Praise
BREATHE HOW YOU WANT TO FEEL

"Matteo's 'tome' on breathwork introduces the reader to a host of new, updated breathwork information that I've never personally discovered in any other breath literature. I highly recommend this read for the library of anyone who wants to optimize their nervous system, better their sleep, and discover clean energy at their beck and call."

— **Ben Greenfield**, *New York Times* best-selling author, biohacker, and physiologist

"Matteo Pistono's insightful book, Breathe How You Want to Feel, *highlights the profound in the simple. He teaches effective and powerful techniques for transforming breathing, the most basic of human functions, into a powerful tool we always have with us that can improve our overall wellness and support the potential of our True Self in coming forward into our lives."*

— **Kimberly Snyder**, *New York Times* best-selling author of *You Are More Than You Think You Are*

"In Breathe How You Want to Feel, *Matteo Pistono weaves ancient wisdom with modern understanding to offer a profound road map for harnessing the transformative power of breath. From the foundational principles to the nuanced practices, Pistono brilliantly guides us to unlock the potential of conscious breathing for personal well-being. This book is a tool kit, a companion to help you navigate life's varied landscapes with mastery over your breath. Whether you seek physiological balance, emotional resilience, or spiritual enrichment, this book is an invaluable guide."*

— **Patrick McKeown**, founder of Buteyko Clinic International and Oxygen Advantage®, author of *The Breathing Cure*

BREATHE HOW YOU WANT TO FEEL

ALSO BY MATTEO PISTONO

In the Shadow of the Buddha: One Man's Journey of Discovery in Tibet

Fearless in Tibet: The Life of the Mystic Tertön Sogyal*

Meditation Made Easy: Coming to Know Your Mind*

Roar: Sulak Sivaraksa and the Path of Socially Engaged Buddhism

*Available from Hay House
Please visit:

Hay House USA: www.hayhouse.com®
Hay House Australia: www.hayhouse.com.au
Hay House UK: www.hayhouse.co.uk
Hay House India: www.hayhouse.co.in

BREATHE HOW YOU WANT TO FEEL

Your Breathing Tool Kit for
Better Health, Restorative Sleep,
and Deeper Connection

MATTEO PISTONO

HAY HOUSE LLC
Carlsbad, California • New York City
London • Sydney • New Delhi

Published in the United States by: Hay House LLC: www.hayhouse.com®
Published in Australia by: Hay House Australia Publishing Pty Ltd: www
.hayhouse.com.au • *Published in the United Kingdom by:* Hay House UK
Ltd: www.hayhouse.co.uk • *Published in India by:* Hay House Publishers
(India) Pvt Ltd: www.hayhouse.co.in

Cover design: Jason Gabbert Design • *Interior design:* Nick C. Welch
Indexer: Shapiro Indexing Services • *Interior illustrations:* Nick C. Welch

Library of Congress Cataloging-in-Publication Data

Tradepaper ISBN: 978-1-4019-7586-9
E-book ISBN: 978-1-4019-7587-6
Audiobook ISBN: 978-1-4019-7588-3

10 9 8 7 6 5 4 3 2 1

1st edition, May 2024

Printed in the United States of America

This product uses responsibly sourced papers and/or recycled materials.
For more information, see www.hayhouse.com.

May every one of us
Breathe how we want to feel,
Breathe how we want to live,
Breathe how we want to die.

CONTENTS

PART III: Breathe How You Want to Die

Scan Me

LISTEN HERE TO FREE
GUIDED BREATHING PRACTICES
BY MATTEO PISTONO

INTRODUCTION

Breath Is Life

Weekends during the late summer and early autumn of my youth were often spent in the mountains of Wyoming with my father and my brother, Mike. We'd usually end our excursions by collecting firewood to take home for our woodstove. On one occasion when I was eight years old, we pulled off South Pass highway onto a dirt road and parked near an outcropping of lodgepole pine. My father cranked the chain saw into action, cutting an old tree that was already on the ground. As my brother stacked the wood in the back of the pickup truck, I explored the forest.

I wandered with my gaze on the forest floor, looking for tracks of the elk and deer that were migrating to lower elevations before the Rocky Mountain winter. We were in a section of dead forest killed by bark beetles. The wind was blowing, and the pine trees were swaying. The trees creaked and cracked. The chain saw buzzing sound was faint as I continued to explore.

A gust of wind blasted through, and I heard a loud crack behind me. I turned to see a 60-foot pine tree falling toward me. I tried to run, but the tree came crashing down. The bark and branches scraped the back of my head, then tore through my flannel shirt and jeans and ripped the skin off my neck, spine, hips, and the backs of my thighs. I whiplashed to the earth. The weight of the tree compressed all the air out of me, pinning me to the ground. With my last breath squeezed out of my chest, my consciousness followed, exiting my body. Suddenly I was floating.

An immediate sense of calmness prevailed. I didn't feel my body. In this suspended state, I drifted toward transparent, concentric halos of light. A soft static sound, like when you try to find a radio station, faded in and out. The tranquility expanded the further I mingled with circles of light. As I hovered into the refractions, I heard my name being called, sounding like an echo from the other side of the valley.

And then, in an instant, the light, floating, and calm vanished. My body burned. My rib cage and chest convulsed me awake, and I was extremely frightened.

"Matt, Matt!" Mike pulled on my arm. I heard the chain saw, and our Labrador, Nick, barking.

I tried to breathe, but I couldn't take in any air. I felt my body trying to breathe me, but the burden of the tree was too great. Face down in the forest turf, I panicked and felt my body seizing. I sniffed, trying to breathe, smelling pine needles.

"Dad! Come here! A tree fell on Matt! Dad!"

My back felt as if it was on fire, my brother was yelling, and then like a candle blown out, everything vanished. Turned off. No lights. No floating. Nothing. Silence.

I don't know how long I was gone; enough time for Mike to run a hundred yards away and gather my father and return to lift the dead tree off me.

When the tree's weight was released, air rushed back into my lungs. Breath and life returned as I opened my eyes.

Twenty-five years after the falling pine tree almost took my life, I found myself sitting next to a Buddhist yogi in a cave in Eastern Tibet. My interest in yoga and Buddhism had taken me from Wyoming to graduate school in London, where I studied Indian philosophy and the Tibetan language, and eventually to Tibet where I sought out teachings. The yogi was instructing me in the esoteric meditation practice known as *tummö,* also known as inner fire practice. The purpose of tummö is to create a psychic heat that rises in the body's central channel and incinerates mental habits of jealousy, pride, and anger, resulting in heightened levels of joy and bliss that evaporate into a nondual state of meditative clarity. The ultimate aim of tummö is nothing short of enlightenment.

I twisted my body into yoga postures as instructed, though it was much different from the yoga classes I had attended in England and the United States. With the yogi observing, I repeatedly elevated myself from a standing position and whipped my legs into full lotus before slamming seated to the ground that sent a shock up my spine. I'd then rotate my head in all directions and rub the energetic meridians of the body with my palms—all while holding my breath for minutes at a time. After a few preliminary rounds of yoga, I'd start tummö, sitting upright while sensing my energetic body as a crystal cylinder and visualizing a flame blazing from just below the navel. Tummö breathing involves slow nasal inhalations, and at the top of the inhalation, I'd swallow and push the air as low as possible. Pulling up on my perineum and pushing my chin onto my sternum, the intra-abdominal pressure of the breath created a vase-like bulging of my belly. The increasing pressure of the breath hold inside my midsection coupled with the intense concentration caused heat to surge throughout my body.

Repeating the slow breathing and holding the vase breath for longer periods of time created waves of bliss-filled delight to well upward through my body. I'd feel the heat moving from my navel throughout my entire body that seemed to flow outward from my crown and fingertips. In the last stage of tummö, there are no breath manipulations, physical movement, or visualizations. Instead, I'd remain motionless and rest in a state of complete openness, not doing anything whatsoever except being panoramically aware of all that arises—while hardly breathing at all.

It wasn't my first time learning esoteric Buddhist practices in Tibet. I'd made frequent pilgrimages to visit holy sites and Tibetan meditation masters in the previous five years, as I was living just south on the other side of the Himalayas in Nepal. I'd moved to Kathmandu after finishing my master's degree in Indian religious-philosophical studies at the School of Oriental and African Studies at the University of London, and I worked on Tibetan cultural programs at the Smithsonian Institution in Washington, D.C. While I loved delving deeply into the study of classic Buddhist philosophy and hatha yoga scriptures in graduate school, I wanted to immerse myself in the actual practices of pranayama, meditation, and tantra. Above all, I wanted to explore the nature of consciousness and learn practices that lead me there. I never forgot the near-death experience when I was eight years old—that liminal state suffused with light where there was no suffering.

Was that breathless but aware state the portal to the other side of death?

Was that the essence of consciousness?

The thread that I found woven through all the Buddhist and hatha yoga practices that lead to the most sublime states of meditation—to the luminous aspect of being—was breath control. I sought teachings from aging meditation masters in Nepal, tantric yogis in Tibet, and wandering ascetics along the Ganges in India. I'd then retreat for weeks and months practicing what they taught me at Buddhist temples in the foothills outside Kathmandu or in hermitages in the mountains of Eastern Tibet. I wanted to extract a lived experience from ancient texts and their practical instructions.

My combined time of meditation retreat lasted more than three years, often secluded and in silence in Nepal, Tibet, India, and Thailand. I wrote several books about these pilgrimages, the solitary time in contemplation, and my encounters, including *In the Shadow of the Buddha*, *Fearless in Tibet*, *Meditation*, and *Roar*. And I began teaching meditation and breathing practices when I returned to the United States.

In my many retreats and still today, when the teachers and gurus stop elaborating, when the yoga postures and prayers conclude, when the mantras fade into silence, it is the breath that leads me into a meditative space of complete openness, effortlessly. There, it feels like consciousness is unbound, free of any boundaries. The breath leads through the portal where thinking and the coarser level of experience dissolve, and the very source of awareness that has no beginning and no end, the centerless center of being, is revealed. This expansive sphere of luminous awareness is where the most subtle aspect of breath and being emerge and dissolve. It is here, a place that has no center or edge, where consciousness is free of duality, that freedom is found, wide open and uncomplicated. With the encouragement of kind teachers and spiritual friends, pilgrims, and yogis, this is the practice that I encountered in Tibet and Nepal and cherish the most today.

This exquisite fusion of breath and awareness, and the flourishing life it offers, is not just for Himalayan hermits, acrobatic yogis, and wise monks and nuns. No, it is for you, me, and every one of us, but we must become an active partner with our breath.

One of my pranayama teachers, David Garrigues, always encourages us to befriend our breath with curiosity, rely on the breath in times of need, wander and play with the breath, and allow it to "open up the vast interior psychological and physical spaces within" our bodies. It is on this journey with the breath that we overcome fear of the unknown, befriend our shadows, face and conquer the inner dragons, and, as Kabir wrote, hear the sounds of "the flute of interior time."[1]

Throughout my more than three decades of study, breath practice, and meditation, I have come to understand that we can breathe how we want to feel, seizing every day so that we can live with no regrets. We can dial up our physiology if we want to become focused, concentrated, and ready for intense or sustained action. On the other hand, we can turn the dial down on our system into restful, calm, and joyful states. Or, with breathing we can balance the energy in our body so that a sky-like meditation is undeniable. Because the way we breathe has such a profound effect on all major systems of the body, and, in particular on our nervous system, harnessing the power of the breath places you in the driver's seat of your emotional, physical, and spiritual well-being.

The state that you are in right now reading this book can be changed with a few conscious breaths. Should you be sleepy right now, you can become attentive with an upregulating breathing pattern. If your mind is racing, you can downregulate into a concentrated state. Should you want to put the book down and fire yourself up for a high-intensity workout, there is a breathing practice for that. If you don't believe me, let's give it a test with this one-minute breathing intervention, the physiological sigh.

PRACTICE

The Physiological Sigh

- Wherever you find yourself right now, sit up comfortably straight. You can do this while walking as well, but not while driving or while in or near water.

- First, bring your attention to your body and let it hover for a few moments to notice the most prominent physical sensations. Just notice your body's sensations.

- Second, move your attention to what thoughts or emotions or feelings are moving through your mind. Again, just notice for a few moments.

- Now, I want you to perform 10 physiological sighs like this: take a full breath in through the nose and hold, pause for a second, and then sniff in so your lungs fill to maximum capacity, and pause momentarily.

- Then exhale out the mouth like you're blowing candles out. So, it's a double inhale, hold for a moment, then a long exhale. No need to rush, but do this 10 times: a full inhale through the nose, a second to top it off, and slowly exhale. Repeat rhythmically for 10 breaths.

- Try it now, and then relax and notice how you feel.

- What do you notice in your body and mind?

I guarantee you feel differently than before, both physically and mentally after that 10-breath intervention.[2] Perhaps more relaxed and at ease mentally? Maybe you feel an energy shift in your body? Take note of the effects of the Physiological Sigh and put it in your breathing tool kit—you'll be adding more throughout the book.

Why I Wrote This Book

The reason I have written *Breathe How You Want to Feel* is to offer you a framework for understanding the profound influence your breathing has on your mental and physical well-being. I want to offer ways for you to harness the power of your breath to take charge of your life rather than being a casualty to life's circumstances. As James Nestor said in *Breath: The New Science of a Lost Art*, "No matter what we eat, how much we exercise, how resilient our genes are, how skinny or young or wise we are—none of it will matter unless we're breathing correctly. That's what these researchers discovered. The missing pillar in health is breath. It all starts there."

As we move through our days, there is an enormous amount of stimulation that leads to chronic stress, repeated anxiety loops, and a lack of command of our emotional world. The anger you felt when the car cut you off in traffic this morning can stay with you for hours. The tension in your jaw or neck you felt when your investments took a hit this afternoon can wake you up in the middle of the night. Stressful situations, people, or even thoughts can exert an incredible power over our emotional well-being. Yet, if you examine your mind, you can see that in between the stimulation around you and your reaction, there is a gap. Viktor Frankl wrote in *Man's Search for Meaning* about his mindset while imprisoned in a Nazi concentration camp, saying, "Between stimulus and response there is a space. In that space is our power to choose our response. In our response lies our growth and our freedom."

We often go through life without recognizing we have a choice in how we want to be, how we want to exist, how we want to feel. Too often, that choice is usurped by our own habitual reactions of volatile temper, jealous pride, and a whole host of other emotions that fuel poor choices in our actions and words, often ones we regret. This book is here to show you how, through the potency of awareness combined with conscious breathing, you no longer will have your power stripped away.

While there are many traditions, protocols, and methods to accomplish this, I'm offering you a three-step strategy of AIR—awareness, intervention, regulation.

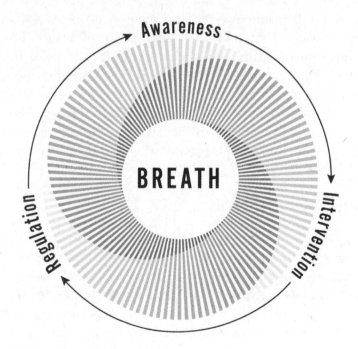

The first step is awareness. To reclaim your power, you must first recognize the dynamism between stressors, your habitual reactions, and how you feel. The second step is a breathing intervention to change your state, to change how you feel. This is not complicated but does need diligence. The third step is regulation, adjusting your breathing throughout the day to sustain how you want to feel. I'm not suggesting that we need to constantly monitor each and every breath and become obsessive—it's a matter of skillfully employing adjustments when needed. AIR is a practical, nondogmatic, and cost-free approach that can be used throughout your life.

While the foundation of AIR is in the philosophy and practices of Buddhism and hatha yoga, what I offer you in this book is not bound to any religion, nor will it be esoteric. It is empowering and requires no belief except in yourself. That said, the consequence of a sustained, conscious breathing practice no doubt can lead you to a numinous portal of spiritual experiences that are beyond words, beyond thoughts, and beyond description. In those moments, I encourage you to simply rest in the expanse of freedom—more on this in the last part of this book when we venture into what is beyond when our breath ceases.

How This Book Is Set Up

Your journey in this book starts with understanding how every single one of the 20,000 breaths you take today build the foundation for your physical, mental, and spiritual well-being. You'll need a breathing tool kit for your journey—this is laid out in Part I. The kit includes the tools of honing your awareness, dialing your nervous system, breathing through your nose, breath holding, and integrating AIR throughout your everyday life. Just as a skilled carpenter applies her tools depending on the job, you will take the five tools and apply them to what you are already doing all day and night: breathing. While you'll learn specific breathing methods and exercises, it is more important that you completely grasp the principles behind the tools and when to use them. In this way you'll be in full control of your breath no matter what life throws at you.

Before each breathing practice, I recommend that you take a moment to think about your intention. This may be a brief thought, such as *May I become more spacious and calmer*, or you might take a bit longer time in contemplation. While I've suggested an intention before each practice, feel free to insert your own, making them meaningful and personal.

Setting an intention before you start is important. It points your heart and mind in the direction you want to go, how you want to be, and perhaps what you want to leave behind. We may have an idea of where we want to arrive and how we want to be with our breathing practice, but if we don't set the intention, our route can be circuitous or miss the mark. Infusing our conscious breathing practice with purpose amplifies its transformative potential.

Part II presents how to use your breathing tool kit in your everyday life. This includes using the breath to jump-start your day, so you don't need to over-caffeinate (though I'd never suggest you shouldn't enjoy your coffee!). You'll learn to breathe optimally when seated at the computer for focus and concentration and before stressful meetings or public speaking. To get the most out of your exercise, there are protocols for how to breathe before your training or workout, during higher-intensity efforts, and for the all-important recovery phase afterward. Whether you are turning up the dials on your system when you want more energy or downregulating your system to enter flow states for meditation and prayer, there are conscious breathing practices. And finally, you'll learn ways to breathe at the end of the day to prepare yourself for taking rest so that your nervous system is primed for restorative sleep. And you'll learn to reduce or stop snoring. The aim of Part II is for your life to flourish.

The theme of Part III may be the most profound. After all that you've learned about breathing interventions, protocols, and methods on changing your immediate state of being, here we talk about letting go. When you release tension in your body and mind, there is no need to brace or clinch any longer. Each exhale is an opportunity to practice letting go of that which is not serving you. Letting go is a profoundly simple practice, yet it's difficult to accomplish. And why should we become skilled in releasing, in truly letting go? Because during the expanse at the end of each exhalation, there is no guarantee that the inhalation will return. Yes, that's correct. Your next breath is not guaranteed.

There is only one thing that is certain in life: that we will die. And there is only one thing certain about our death: we don't know when it will occur. Contemplating our mortality, even practicing our own death, is not morbid or depressing. To the contrary, daily remembrance of our own mortality has the power to bring into sharp clarity what is most important in life. All that we have in life exists, and then passes, so that its preciousness can be known. We let go with each exhalation into this realization, with gratitude. Contemplating death makes our priorities clear. Practicing dying brings confidence in life. There is no time like right now to prepare for that unknown time. So, while there are times when we need to intervene and change the way we breathe so that we can thrive, we also need to learn to let go, appreciate with gratitude, and recognize the ever-changing flow of experience, right here, right now. We practice this in the last part of the book.

There are a variety of breathing practices and exercises throughout the book. The practices are designed so that you gain an experiential understanding of how the different ways that you inhale, exhale, and hold your breath impact your physiology and how you feel. All the practices can be done in standalone breathing sessions or spontaneously throughout the day, and I encourage you to work with them over the course of days and months. By the end of this book, you'll have a firm grasp on breathing mechanics and physiology, which empowers you with resilience and confidence.

All the practices in *Breathe How You Want to Feel* are bolstered by evidence-based research from pulmonologists, neurologists, and behavioral biologists and show how optimal breathing can positively impact your brain function, cardiovascular strength, and mental health. We'll also gather encouragement from the current wave of experts incorporating breathing for human performance from the communities of Oxygen Advantage, the Health & Human Performance Foundation, XPT Extreme Performance Training, and others, inspiring us to reach our full potential. And finally, we take inspiration from pulmonautic pioneers who explored what is in between and beyond the breath itself.

It is my sincere wish that you can extract from this book an experiential understanding of the power of your breath, one that moves within you with every inhale and exhale. I want you to breathe optimally so that your life flourishes mentally, physically, and spiritually—so that you can breathe how you want to feel, breathe how you want to live, and breathe how you want to die. May your breath bestow upon you all the blessings and power that you are seeking and may any benefit ripple out to your family, community, and beyond.

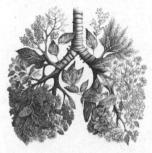

Part I

THE
5 PRINCIPLES
OF OPTIMAL
BREATHING

Chapter 1

BREATH IS THE MOST FUNDAMENTAL ASPECT OF YOUR BEING

Whether you are aware of your breath or not, breathing happens automatically. If you live beyond the age of 80, you'll breathe close to a billion breaths in your lifetime—a billion! Today alone you'll breathe 20,000 times, and of those, how many breaths will you be aware of? Really, how many breaths will you watch come in and go out?

Have you observed today how your inhalation is slightly cool around your nostrils, how your abdomen or torso move, or if there is a slight pause before the exhalation? Did you notice today when you unconsciously held your breath while scrolling on your phone? Are your lips and mouth dry because you are breathing through your mouth? Did you take note when your breathing felt shallow and up in your chest and how that affected your emotions? Or did it occur to you how your breathing contributed to how well rested you felt this morning when you woke up? If you have poor digestion, lower-back pain, sexual dysfunction, or brain fog, did you consider the role your breathing mechanics play in those aliments?

I've been asked innumerable times, "If I breathe automatically, why should I change anything?"

Just because you breathe automatically doesn't mean you breathe optimally—and breathing optimally allows you to breathe how you want to feel. If you are stressed, anxious, or fearful, as all of us are at times and to varying degrees, if you don't control your breath, your breath will control you.

We all breathe differently. Some of us breathe primarily through the nose; others are mouth breathers. Some take slow breaths with the diaphragm doing most of the respiratory work. Others breathe rapidly and use their neck and upper-chest muscles. Some breaths are smooth while others are halting on the way in and stutter on the way out. Some breaths make wheezing noises while others are silent. There are a thousand other ways to describe the simple act of breathing—indeed no two breaths are the same!

All the different ways that we breathe directly impact how we feel, and the way we feel impacts how we breathe—it's a two-way street. Some ways of breathing might be called optimal and others suboptimal, and we're going to explore what works best for you.

Optimal and Suboptimal Breathing

Optimal breathing refers to a breathing pattern that promotes good health, well-being, and performance, both physically and mentally. Breathing optimally during your normal day involves a combination of three principal factors that include breathing through the nose, using the diaphragm and rib muscles to breathe, and maintaining a slow and flowing breathing rhythm.

Suboptimal breathing refers to chronic mouth breathing, taking shallow breaths, breathing rapidly, or breathing in other ways that do not support your body and mind. There is a cascade of negative physical and mental health consequences when you do not breathe optimally. Specific to your physiology, your nervous system is thrown out of balance, which leads to poor sleep, a decrease in heart rate variability, and an increased level of stress hormones and anxiety levels. In turn, this can cause fatigue, difficulty concentrating, depression, and other psychological issues and long-term physical ailments.

The ways we breathe are influenced by various internal and external factors in our lives. Traumatic events, chronic stress, and worry can trigger the body's "fight, flight, or freeze" response, leading us to brace ourselves against the world and hold the belly and chest tense, like having a tight emotional corset. And the clothes we wear—such as tight trousers, belts, and skirts—can restrict our breathing. Societal influences impact us; I recall being told by my grade school teacher, "Hold your belly in!" Modern sedentary lifestyles; excessive screen time; and prolonged hours spent sitting in cars, chairs, trains, and in front of computers all contribute to altering the natural open and flowing nature of our breath. Older age and physical injuries can also result in suboptimal breathing patterns. These cumulative factors have disrupted the innate harmony and ease of the simple rhythmic action of our breath.

The primary factors contributing to suboptimal breathing among a majority of adults and teenagers in the U.S. and U.K. are twofold.[1] First, there are issues related to poor breathing mechanics, such as habitual mouth breathing, excessive use of the upper chest instead of the diaphragm, and unconscious breath holding. Second, psychological disturbances, including stress-induced breathing dysfunction, also play a significant role. In many cases, these factors can interact and combine to contribute to the problem.

The good news is that it is not difficult to learn, or relearn, proper mechanics to breathe optimally. When you breathe optimally, you can regulate your nervous system. Knowing how to regulate your own nervous system is nothing other than a secret power. The efforts you make in changing how you breathe optimally have exponential positive effects on your energy levels and mood enhancement, emotions, sleep quality, and the quality of your personal life, including relationships.

Breathing optimally doesn't mean always breathing calmly. Instead, breathing optimally is breathing in a manner that is congruent with the way we want to feel in whatever activity we are engaged in. Some breathing exercises stimulate and wake you up, which are good to do in the morning or afternoon but not before bed. Other breathing interventions relax you deeply, which are not usually appropriate first thing in the morning. While there are general breathing intervention guidelines I'll offer you, please be playful and experimental with your breath. Your curiosity in your breath leads to deeper self-awareness and ability to self-regulate. As Dr. Peter Attia writes in *Outlive: The Science and Art of Longevity,* "The way in which we breathe reflects how we interact with the world."[2]

If you are reading or listening to this book, chances are high that you have already encountered the power of conscious breathing, whether in a yoga class, associated with a meditation practice, or if your partner or a friend said, "Take a deep breath." Perhaps your friend told you how a relaxing breath pattern improved their sleep. Maybe your doctor recommended "Belly Breathing" to calm you down before bed or when you were recovering from a surgery. Best-selling books like James Nestor's *Breath* demonstrate the immense interest in breathing. Stories abound of elite athletes, from NBA and MLB players to big-wave surfers to Olympians using conscious breathing to control their adrenaline, maintain focus, and relax when needed. The mounting medical and scientific research around the world into the efficacy of the entire spectrum of therapeutic breathing protocols is at an all-time high.[3]

The Blessed Breath

There are several ways to understand the primacy of the breath for our well-being. Let's consider the spiritual perspective first.

The breath is at the foundation of many religions around the world. The Abrahamic religions of Judaism, Christianity, and Islam are united in the belief that breathing is a sacred act. The Hebrew word *ruach* has a dual meaning of "breath" and "spirit of life," and we see in the Torah that "the spirit of God formed me; the breath of the Almighty sustains me." In the Bible it states, "Then the Lord God formed a man from the dust of the ground and breathed into his nostrils the breath of life, and the man became a living being." The Koran similarly mentions divine breath multiple times, including, "I will bring into being a human being out of dry ringing clay . . . When I have completed shaping him and breathed into him of My Spirit." Breath in the Torah, Bible, and Koran is nothing other than the power of God animating humanity.[4]

We see in each of these traditions how later practitioners used the breath to deepen their spiritual practice. Shortly following Christ's resurrection, he appeared to his disciples, breathing upon them and uttering the words "receive the Holy Spirit."[5] This act is later symbolically reenacted within the Christian sacrament of baptism, where, in some traditions, the priest imparts the Holy Spirit by blowing upon the acolyte. St. Augustine's now-famous prayer invokes the Holy Spirit to "breathe in me," and four centuries later, Coptic Christians, such as St. John Klimakos, added practices of coordinating the rhythm of breathing with the invocation of the Holy Name, "Let the remembrance of Jesus be united with your breathing." By the 14th century, the Hesychast monks, who some have called "Byzantine yogis," used bodily postures, Cadence Breathing, and breath holds to lead the seeker away from the intellect and into the heart to affirm, "Jesus is invoked with every breath." This is similar to the Sufi practice of *dhikr*—the remembrance and invoking the name of God—repeating different syllables upon the inhalation and exhalation of the breath.

The most comprehensive breathing practices ever developed arose in the yogic traditions from the Indian sub-continent, which we know today as pranayama. The word *pranayama* is a Sanskrit compound, with *prana* meaning "life force" or "vitality" and *ayama* meaning "extension" or, in some cases, "restraint" of the breath (e.g., breath holding). Extending, manipulating, and retaining one's prana is accomplished through mastering control of the three phases of breathing—inhalation, exhalation, and the pauses between. Innumerable pranayama techniques were developed by controlling these three phases. In the minds of yogis and philosophers in ancient India, as evident in the vast corpus of scriptures, breathing signified life and what humans breathed was the driving energy behind the universe itself.[6] The cosmic wind is mankind's vital breath (prana), the principal manifestation of his immortal soul. The many traditions and religions of the Indian subcontinent—Zoroastrian, Hindu, Buddhist, Jain, and Sikh—were all in robust debate and self-experiments, especially during the Vedic period, about how to fulfill their spiritual pursuits with the power of the breath.

The historical Buddha likely practiced pranayama during his six years of austerities before his enlightenment under the Bodhi tree. But there is no evidence that he taught these yogic breathing practices during his 45 years of teaching. Instead, the Buddha emphasized the fundamental "breath awareness" practice, instructing his disciples not to change the way they breathed but rather place their mind upon the breath and mindfully observe its ebb and flow. If the breath was long and slow, watch the breath be long and slow. If it was short and fast, witness that pace. He used the breath as an anchor for concentration. When the concentrated mind was distracted, the Buddha taught mindfulness as a method to return the mind back to its chosen object of concentration. The principle aim of mindfulness practice is to develop single pointed concentration, a necessary function of the mind applied to latter practices of investigating the nature of consciousness.

Why didn't the Buddha teach his students to manipulate the breath, or in our modern language, to upregulate or downregulate the nervous system with breathing practices like the ones explored in this book? It should be remembered who the Buddha was teaching: renunciate monks and nuns who did not have the chronic stressors or wave after wave of digital distractions of today. His disciples were psychologically regulated and well positioned to simply observe the breath with no need to downregulate an overly stimulated nervous system.

In the centuries after the Buddha passed into nirvana some 2,500 years ago, there was a resurgence in pranayama with the rise of tantric practices among Buddhists and Hindus—and there was cross-pollination between practices and lineages. Breath control was combined with many different yogic postures, mantra recitation, visualizations, and breath holds while performing "energetic locks" at the perineum, navel, and chin. The purpose of these yogic pranayama practices is to stimulate and preserve vital essence within the body and redirect it for spiritual attainments.[7]

Mastery of breath holds, or *kumbhaka*, was the key to physical yoga for these yogis. In contrast to today's yoga at your local studio, where the focus is on acrobatic body postures or simply stretching, the defining characteristic of classical hatha yoga is breath control. When you control your breath, you have the power to navigate skillfully your internal mental, emotional, and spiritual landscape with ease. Along with the tantric notion that the body was a microcosm of the universe, a defining characteristic of the teachings from this time was that the mind cannot be controlled by the mind, but only by the breath.

Controlling one's breath as a cornerstone of the spiritual path flourished throughout the Indian subcontinent and traveled with Buddhism and Tantra over the Himalayas into Tibet. Tibetan Buddhist yogis developed pranayama in their tantric subtle body practices. These esoteric practices taught ways to increase vital essences of the body and redistribute them into the energetic centers along their central axis to intensify experience of nonconceptual bliss.

Maps of Understanding the Breath

I've gained much by studying the techniques, methods, and metaphysical frameworks of different religious traditions to understand consciousness and breathing. I appreciate that each tradition offers their own map of understanding. A map of understanding is a way of organizing vast amounts of knowledge in a structured manner, so students gain a deeper understanding of complex concepts. Such maps of understanding are used not only among spiritual traditions but also in philosophy and psychology.

The Abrahamic maps connect our breath with the God-given soul, and associated liturgies and prayers have developed from there. Hindu and tantric maps of understanding use the breath and prana to cleanse and energize the body's meridians and chakras, sometimes adding imagery of coiled snakelike energy at the base of the spine, ready to surge upward with the breath and bring waves of bliss. Buddhists have their variety of maps of understanding across the different traditions, including Vajrayana maps that teach how to use the breath to guide your consciousness out of the body at the time of death.

There are hundreds of other maps of understanding across the worldwide spiritual landscape—from ancient Egypt to the Aztec Empire, from Qigong masters of China to the Kalahari, from Kung Bushmen to the Plains Indian of the Great Basin in North America—showing how to use the breath for spiritual aims. All of them point to the breath as the most fundamental aspect of being. And any of us can use these maps of understanding if we find them helpful in our development of physical, mental, and spiritual health.

While religious and spiritual traditions all have recognized the power of the breath, no tradition can claim ultimate authority on the breath. This is important to recognize because the power of the breath, *the power of your breath*, resides within you, and not within a tradition, a saint, or a guru. It is for you to gain an experiential understanding of the sanctity and power of your breath.

Your Autonomic Nervous System

The map of understanding that we'll use mostly in *Breathe How You Want to Feel* comes from modern physiology. This map presents how your central nervous system runs the functioning of your body and is involved with every aspect of your health. The command center for your nervous system, according to this map, is the brain and spinal column, which is responsible for all your major organ functions, your sleep and waking cycles, digestion, and breathing, as well as the mental sphere of perception, thinking, memory, and feeling emotions.

A key part of the central nervous system is the autonomic system. Your autonomic nervous system communicates to and takes orders from the brain to run your body—including your blood pressure, heart and breathing rate, digestion, body temperature, production of saliva and sweat, excretion, and sexual functions. If your central nervous system is the command center, the autonomic system are the dutiful legions (nerve cells) communicating from the landscape of your body. This system is called autonomic because it happens autonomously without your conscious effort.

To understand the role your breath plays in your nervous system, it's important to differentiate the two divisions of the autonomic nervous system—the sympathetic and parasympathetic nervous systems. These two systems work in tandem to regulate various physiological processes and maintain balance in the body.

AUTONOMIC NERVOUS SYSTEM

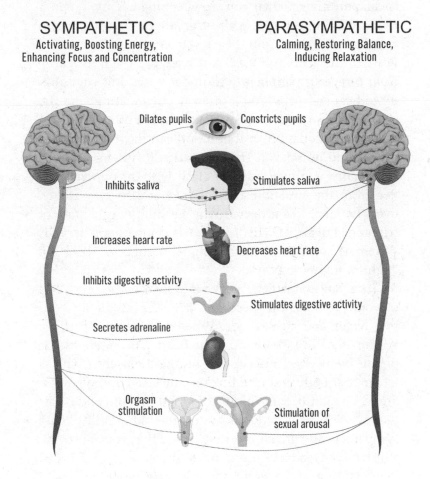

The sympathetic nervous system is responsible for your aroused, energetic, and sometimes stressful mental and physical states. This is when stress hormones are released, and your body is flooded with cortisol, adrenaline, and noradrenaline. When your sympathetic nervous system is active, you feel an increasing and concentrated energy in the body and mind.

Think of when you are about to begin a competitive game of football or soccer or perhaps right before you speak publicly, or when you are watching a scary movie—that provoked feeling is your sympathetic nervous system kicking into gear. Your heart rate increases and blood flows to the arms and legs, as if readying them for battle or to run. Your peripheral vision decreases, but your ability to hear sharpens. You'll often begin sweating, and the signals in your body to urinate are turned off. Your digestion also switches off so that blood can move to the vital organs and muscles. If the sympathetic system responds maximally, you may want to clash with an opponent or flee from the situation altogether. You also may freeze, overwhelmed, like a deer in the headlights in a state of frightened disbelief. This is why the sympathetic nervous system is sometimes called "fight, flight, or freeze" or "fight-or-flight" response.

The parasympathetic nervous system is the other end of your physiological spectrum. It is responsible for your rest, repair, and digest mode. When your parasympathetic system is more prominent, your heart rate lowers as the organs prepare to conserve and restore themselves. This is when your body and mind relax. Salivation and digestion are ready to utilize nutrition from food to build and repair tissues. With your body and mind relaxed and not being sympathetically driven, stressed, or reactive, you are able to think more creatively and manage situations with a broad view. During the parasympathetic state, your body and mind adapt to previously stressful situations, high learning is assimilated, and neural plasticity is at its highest.

Throughout the day, your autonomic nervous system vacillates between different degrees of sympathetic and parasympathetic tone. Human physiology, like nearly all the animal kingdom, evolved in this manner so that it can upregulate in high-demand situations and survive and downregulate when the threat has passed so a person can recover, digest food, and relax enough to have sex. A healthy nervous system can toggle between the two tones as needed and appropriate, without becoming too lethargic or too stressed. The autonomic nervous system at its most fundamental design evolved for survival and procreation. And while it functions automatically, you can intercede and consciously control it—with your breath.

Before surfing or higher-intensity exercise, I upregulate my nervous system into sympathetic dominance with a five-minute moderately intensive conscious breathing practice with a few rounds of fast-paced, diaphragmatic bellows-like breathing. My heart rate increases, digestion turns off, and adrenal glands are stimulated but not so much so that it moves me into a fully stressed situation. I want blood flow to increase to my arms to paddle, and I want some adrenaline in the body and brain as I enter in the ocean focused for the challenge.

On the other hand, when I sit down to eat a dinner with my wife, I consciously extend my exhalations for 5 to 10 breaths to elicit a parasympathetic response. I breathe until I feel sweet saliva develop in my mouth, and I know blood is flowing into my digestive tract, ensuring healthy digestion. It also calms my mind so I'm completely present with my family.

Your Breathing Tool Kit

In any life situation, the fastest way to shift your physiology, to change your state, is to breathe in a manner that regulates your sympathetic or parasympathetic nervous systems. Conscious breathing is accessible to everyone, is a zero-cost tool, and is proven effective. As Dr. Andrew Weil, the grandfather of integrative medicine, said over two decades ago, "Of all the techniques that I have investigated for reducing stress and increasing relaxation, it is breathwork that I have found to be the most time-efficient, the most cost-effective, and the one that most promotes increased wellness and optimal health."[8]

In the next five chapters, you'll assemble your breathing tool kit, which will include:

- Cultivating awareness

- Adjusting the dials on your nervous system

- Breathing through your nose

- Holding your breath consciously

- Integrating AIR (awareness, intervention, and regulation)

You don't need complicated methods and techniques, pricey retreats or seminars, or a new belief system or metaphysical notions. Rather, you only need to apply a few principles from your breathing tool kit to what you are already doing 20,000 times a day. This isn't a lifestyle hack—it is optimizing the most fundamental aspect of your existence, your breath, into all aspects of your life.

KEY INSIGHTS

- While breathing is automatic, you have the power to alter your breathing to change your state, to breathe how you want to feel. Each inhalation and exhalation affects your well-being. Awareness of the breath is the starting point: use breathing interventions when needed and regulation throughout the day—this is AIR.

- When we become aware of the space between stimulation (from the world around us and our thoughts) and our response, we regain power in our lives. Rather than reacting habitually and unconsciously, we respond appropriately. Your personal power lies in your awareness and control of your breath.

- You can consciously self-regulate your autonomic nervous system with your breath, shifting as needed between the aroused sympathetic nervous system for alert and physically demanding states to the relaxed, parasympathetic response for times of recovery and digestion. You have the power.

Chapter 2

CULTIVATING AWARENESS

Your ability to breathe how you want to feel, to regulate your nervous system, begins with awareness. Awareness is the first step of our AIR strategy—awareness, intervention, and regulation. In the beginning of your efforts to use the breath to empower you, it's necessary to be diligent in your awareness. This is because habitual tendencies of dysfunctional breathing are often strong and deeply entrenched. Your diligence is rewarded within days when the benefits reaped from optimal breathing are a reminder itself to keep up the practice. Eventually, your breathing mechanics and biochemistry upgrade to such a degree that your physiology adapts to become more efficient. But your breathing mechanics and biochemistry need consistent training.

Let's define awareness. Awareness is the knowing quality of your mind. It is that part of your being that knows what is perceived by way of your five senses—seeing, hearing, tasting, touching, and smelling—as well as your thoughts and emotions. Being aware of the flow of life around and within you may sound simple. But it is a challenge, especially in today's world, where there is unceasing competition for your attention from social media, advertisements, politicians, news, and entertainment. We may spend hour upon hour scrolling, clicking between messages and websites, watching TV, jumping between audiobooks, news, and podcasts; our world becomes an endless stream of distractions from the life that is around us. Our awareness is fragmented.

There is an illusion that we can autonomously choose where to direct our awareness—this is not the case for most of us. Rather, with outside influences driving our attention, we live our days in a reactive mode, steered by the latest post, video, or talking head. This reactive mode is laced with tension because what we see on screens and entertainment all too often fuels a sense of inadequacy, a lack of self-worth, and dependence on external validation. I write this knowing this has also been the case for me, and nearly everyone I know.

As if it was not difficult enough to have our attention highjacked by the media and screens, we also must tend with the surge of stimulation that comes from within our minds in the form of thoughts and emotions. Everyone experiences thought loops where we can't seem to stop ruminating on something that bothers us. These repetitive thought patterns cause chronic stress during the day, keep us from falling asleep, and awaken us in the middle of the night. Feedback loops between thoughts and our stressful reaction reinforces worry and the increasing degree of felt anxiety. The feedback loop disempowers our ability to manage not only our thinking but also our emotions, energy, and behavior, holding us back from taking care of ourselves and those around us. There is no self-regulation when we are in a constant fragmented and reactive state.

Whether distraction and disempowerment come from outside or from within, the first step to reclaiming your autonomy is being aware that this process is happening. Without this initial spark of awareness, there is no course correction. Instead, we are bound to our distractions, cyclical thought loops, habitual reactions, and the mental and physical angst that ensues. But with awareness, we intercede and cut the usual reaction. Instead of reacting habitually, we respond consciously by taking control of our nervous system to change our state. As Dr. Elissa Epel encourages us in *The Stress Prescription,* let stress be a reminder to become resilient.[1]

Initiating a Breathing Intervention

How do we change our state right now? By initiating conscious breath control. Intervention is the second step of the AIR strategy—awareness, intervention, regulation. Initiating conscious breathing provides a pattern interrupt, which is a technique used in meditation and cognitive psychology to shift the mind away from its habitual patterns of thought, to get you out of the mental grooves that seem intractable. Pattern interruption involves introducing a different stimulus to an existing mental pattern to disrupt it and create opportunity for fresh insight. This technique breaks through blockages that keep you entrenched in negative self-talk, anxiety, or other unhelpful mental habits.

When you initiate a conscious breathing pattern, you position your awareness to observe what is actually happening within you and watch real-time changes. If you try to only engage your mental faculties without the somatic assistance of the breath, as I have seen repeatedly with many meditators who try to think themselves out of stressful situations, the thinking mind is too emotionally clouded to see clearly. This is to say, it is extremely difficult, if not impossible, to think yourself out of a stressful situation. Rather, using the breath to tap in to your internal awareness with a nonjudgmental perspective affords you the space to become cognizant of the various physical and emotional components of any experience.

Mantra, prayer, or positive self-talk are all options to use as pattern interruptions, but they still rely on the mind (or beliefs) to overcome emotions—and this is a tall order. The advantage of using the breath as a pattern interrupter is that your physiology is changed within moments, and we often need that immediate support. A breathing intervention creates a brief pause in your sympathetic nervous system's response. During this pause, you can feel and connect with a sense of spaciousness, and this allows the dark emotional clouds that are obscuring the sky-like clarity of your awareness to clear. In other words, with your breath, you gain some control over your nervous system's threat response. Conscious breathing is the quickest and most certain way to change your psychological state because, as research has demonstrated, breathing interventions constitute a potent avenue to manipulate the whole physiological state.[2]

That said, it is important to recognize the limitations of conscious breathing interventions when acute psychological states happen, such as full-blown panic or manic episodes. Attempting breathing interventions during an actual panic attack may not be helpful and can exacerbate the episode. Instead, it is advisable to incorporate conscious breathing into your daily routine when you are feeling grounded. By doing so, you can practice conscious breathing for when those moments of overwhelming anxiety happen. Additionally, when conscious slow breathing, along with other modalities that help you self-regulate, is regularly done, it can have a significant impact on reducing the frequency and intensity of panic attacks. The key is to practice de-escalation techniques— parasympathetic nervous system activation—when you are feeling well so you increase your resilience when stressors hit. Once you feel comfortable with the breathing interventions, you can experiment with incorporating long, slow breaths or other interventions when you feel anxiety levels rising. This approach may interrupt the progression toward a full-blown attack and allow you to be fully present with the emotional and physical aspects of what you are experiencing.

Developing Your Interoception with Breath Awareness

Tapping into awareness of your psychosomatic state is what neuroscientists call *interoception*. Interoception is the awareness of internal bodily sensations and its associated feelings and emotions. Interoception is not the examination or observation of your mental and emotional process; that's *introspection*. Rather, interoception involves the ability to sense and interpret signals from your internal organs and physiological systems, and to respond appropriately.

The most fundamental way to recognize your interoceptive awareness is when you feel hunger or thirst, physical pain, a sense of being tired or awake, or when you have to go to the bathroom—observing this process is instructive in understanding the impact the physical has on how you feel, and vice versa. We can develop a more subtle interoceptive awareness of both the sensations inside our body and our autonomic nervous system as it impacts our emotional state. For example, when we initiate a relaxing breath pattern, the feeling of calm is known by our interoception.[3]

Interoception is your internal compass that guides you to recognize the shifting landscape within your body and mind. When skillful at using this compass, we're better able to recognize and manage our emotions, to identify physiological cues of stress and implement coping strategies, and to make better decisions.

In the absence of interoceptive awareness, messages from your body may go unnoticed, leading to dulled perceptions. Interoceptive receptors serve as vital conduits, transmitting internal body information to the discerning brain. Insufficient interoception renders you more susceptible to being stirred by internal stressors—be it the tumult of thoughts or the turbulence of emotions—as well as the reverberations of external stress on your well-being. Such limitations in interoception can breed irritability, manifesting in instances where even trivial disturbances, like a misplaced object or a minor delay, trigger an exaggerated response.

Interoceptive awareness is improved through various practices, including yoga, tai chi, mindfulness, and meditation, but in my experience and the observations of others, breath awareness is the place to start for sharpening your interoception. The reason for this is because recognizing how you feel and how your breathing pattern is presenting itself establishes a baseline. After your breathing intervention, being aware of how you feel offers you critical information as to the efficacy of what you just did; in other words, did changing your breathing make you feel the way you want?

But it starts with breath awareness. In breath awareness practice, there is no control or manipulation of your breath. You merely point the spotlight of your attention fully on the ebb and flow of breathing in whichever way the breath is showing up. If your breath is long and slow, you notice that and how that makes you feel. If the breath is halting and shallow, you notice that and how that makes you feel. Noticing how your breath is presenting itself and how you feel in any moment is your baseline—this is breath awareness.

Like when you sit still next to a river and listen deeply, your open attentiveness reveals many layers of sounds. Trickling, gurgling, whooshing—all flowing in and out of each other. Similarly, with breath awareness practice, you listen, feel, and observe the many layers of your breath as it moves in and through you.

Breath awareness practice involves a key principle: *allowing the breath to breathe you.* Allowing the breath to breathe you means becoming the witness to your breath. There is no manipulation or breathing intervention in breath awareness practice. Instead, you cultivate a state of nonjudgmental observation of the breath and notice how you feel. Should you want to change how you feel, the next step is breathing intervention.

Let's practice letting the breath breathe you. And just a note before the practice: when you fix your attention on the breath initially, you may notice that you exert some control, such as breathing deeper or exhaling longer—this is normal. When that initial controlling is noticed, attempt to relax, and adopt a witnessing mode of attention toward your breath. Let go. Allow the breath to breathe you.

PRACTICE

Allowing the Breath to Breathe You

- Find a comfortable position while seated, lying down, or walking.

- Take a moment to remind yourself why you are turning your attention toward your breath, perhaps thinking: *Through breath awareness, may I cultivate a spacious and generous attitude.*

- Take a few moments to notice how your body feels, and notice what is happening in your mind.

- Turn your attention to your breath. No need to change anything, just observe the breath. If you'd like to have a hand on your belly for somatic feedback, that is fine.

- You may notice some control that you are exerting over your inhale or exhale. Slowly relax and let go.

- Relax your eyes and temples and your neck and shoulders, and let your belly be loose.

- Allow your breath to breathe you.

- Breathe in and out of your nose.

- Notice wherever you feel the breath most prominently—either around your nostril, the belly, or somewhere else. Once you feel the breath movement, let your attention settle there.

- Maintain a relaxed attentiveness—not too tight, and not too loose.

- Observe the inhale, the slight pause at the top, and the exhalation, and the slight pause at the bottom.

- How is your inhalation? Cool or warm? Smooth or stuttering? Short or long? Just observe. There is no need to change anything.

- How is your exhalation? Flowing or does it stairstep out? Is there anticipation for something beyond the exhale?

- What happens in between breaths?

- Is the breath full? Is there a physical feeling of breathlessness?

- Just observe whatever is presenting itself as you breathe in and as you breathe out.

- There may be emotions rising—no need to push them away or ruminate on them. Just observe.

- If your mind wanders and begins to think about something else, this is normal. When you notice, release the thoughts, relax your body, and return to the breath—each time, release, relax, return.

- Watch the inhale come in. Watch the exhale go out. And observe the spaces in between.

- Allow your breath to breathe you.

- Continue for 5 to 10 minutes or for however long you feel fresh.

- At the conclusion, let go of watching your breath and notice for a minute or so how your body and mind feel.

You can practice breath awareness in a formal session, like a meditation practice, or it can be spontaneous. In both cases, cultivating breath awareness improves your interoception. Then you can choose if you want to change your state by initiating a breathing intervention.

To help you plan, it might be helpful to decide right now where you'll rest your awareness when you want to take a moment for breath awareness. Perhaps you'll direct your attention to the feeling of cool air entering your nostrils or the feedback of your hand on your belly, or maybe you'll rest your awareness in the pause at the end of the exhalation. As many Buddhist meditation teachers advise, practice breath awareness in "short sessions, many times." Directing your awareness for one inhalation and exhalation is a "session," though if you want to continue for 5 or 10 minutes, that is great as well. It is more beneficial to practice breath awareness 10 times a day for a few refreshing breaths than it is to doze in and out of sleep during a 20-minute meditation session!

The Long Road to the Zafu

After checking in with breath awareness, if you want to change how you feel, the second step of AIR is to initiate your breathing intervention. This is a crucial step that takes diligence. You can know a bunch of different breathing techniques and have all the knowledge about the nervous system, but if this step from awareness to intervention is not taken, then all that knowledge is wasted.

The gap between knowing and doing has long been a struggle in meditation traditions and is sometimes called "the long road to the zafu." A zafu is a meditation cushion in the Zen tradition. Often when a meditator knows it's time to sit on the zafu to meditate, procrastination sets in. They'll decide to rearrange or clean the room, then maybe fix a cup of tea or coffee or light another stick of incense. In today's world, perhaps they even scroll their phone to check on a to-do list, finding various other things that keep them from just sitting down to meditate. The long road to the zafu is the main reason so many people have meditation apps but never meditate. We might remember what Leonardo da Vinci said: "I have been impressed with the urgency of doing. Knowing is not enough; we must apply. Being willing is not enough; we must do."

Once you've checked in with breath awareness, initiate a breath practice there and then—there is no reason to delay.

What breathing intervention should you initiate? That is exactly what you are going to learn in the next chapter by familiarizing yourself with different interventions that adjust the dials on your nervous system. One size does not fit all when it comes to breathing. It is important to know the dials on your nervous system so you can self-regulate—the third step of AIR. So, let's dive into the next tool in your breathing tool kit—the breathing dials on your nervous system.

KEY INSIGHTS

- Awareness is the key that opens the door to the benefits of conscious breathing practice. Breathing how you want to feel begins with recognizing your internal state and then applying an intervention.

- The quickest way to change your state, to intervene in your physiology, is by controlling your breath.

- The best time to breathe how you want to feel is right now—no need to delay.

Chapter 3

ADJUSTING THE DIALS ON YOUR NERVOUS SYSTEM

You can consciously control your sympathetic and parasympathetic nervous systems with how you breathe. Remember, your sympathetic nervous system is responsible for being ready for action, being physically and mentally alert, focused, and energized. Your parasympathetic nervous system mellows you out, turning on your digestion and allowing you to rest and recharge. These two systems work in concert with each other, and you can turn them up or down with different breathing dials.

The three main breathing dials you have are:

The strength of your breath—light to powerful

The pace of your breath—slow to quick

The depth of your breath—shallow to deep

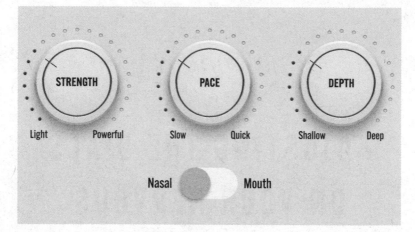

Like an old-school boom box or a music producer's dials on a mixing board with different levels of bass, treble, and volume for the perfect sound, you adjust the dials on your nervous system for how you want to feel. You can turn all three dials or toggle between mouth or nasal breathing, depending on your desired effects. We'll discuss extensively the physiological effects of nasal versus mouth breathing later. But let's get right into the three breathing dials now.

The First Dial: Strength of Your Breath— Light to Powerful

The strength or exertion of how you breathe immediately affects how you feel in body and mind. Take three very powerful inhales and exhales right now . . . go ahead and do it. Strong inhale. Strong exhale. Again. And a third time. Then release and notice.

You likely feel a surge of energy, your heart rate increased, you might feel heat in your face and around your ears and perhaps tingling in your hands—you just turned the strength dial on the sympathetic nervous system.

The strength that you breathe, from very light where you can barely feel the hairs moving in your nostrils to very powerful where you are huffing and puffing through your mouth or nose, affects the delivery of oxygen throughout the body. We'll discuss in the next chapter the optimal way to breathe for maximal uptake of oxygen into your brain and cells (spoiler alert: despite the popular but mistaken notion that big, heavy breathing delivers more oxygen, light, slow nasal breaths are the way to go!), but to understand the dials on the nervous system, you have the option to move the breath lightly or powerfully either through the nose or mouth.

There are situations when it's beneficial to move the breath in a very forceful manner—for example, if you need to sprint a short distance when your young child wanders into the street, right before you lift a heavy object, or if you have to evade a wild animal. When you take a couple of strong breaths, your sympathetic nervous system spikes immediately and will increase as you continue to breathe powerfully. Powerful breathing causes your adrenal glands to release stress hormones called adrenaline (epinephrine) and cortisol, which causes blood to surge to your arms and legs, readying them for action; increases your heart rate; and dilates the pupils of your eyes to assess for threats on the periphery. Mentally stressful situations such as an argument with a loved one or unexpected terrible news can also cause you to increase the strength of the breath, moving you into a fight-or-flight mode. If you continue to breathe forcefully, either from physical exertion or feelings of panic, hyperventilation can ensue with the associated lightheadedness, weakness, confusion, and muscle spasms, and possibly fainting.

The use of powerful breaths is beneficial in unique circumstances when there is a specific call to action. For example, when a firefighter is racing up a burning stairwell to save a child or other circumstances that demand immediate response to danger and threats. Our ability to respond to stressful situations at a moment's notice is truly remarkable—and a healthy physiology allows for that when needed. But unless you are involved in high-demand situations, chances are slim that you regularly need to breathe to spike your sympathetic nervous system with heavy breathing. In fact, if you do chronically breathe in a way that causes your body and mind to swim day and night in stress hormones, the consequences are dire. As Dr. Epel and other stress researchers emphasize, "Chronic stress doesn't do anything good for you. It's only damaging."[1]

The litany of health ramifications from chronic stress includes risk of obesity, heart disease, diabetes, depression, and dementia. And in the short-term, mental effects of stress can include anxiety, irritability, and low self-esteem. The physical consequences may manifest as fatigue and low energy, frequent headaches, sexual dysfunction, and poor sleep and digestion.

While we don't want to breathe throughout the day in a way that strains our nervous system, there are certain conscious breathing practices whose purpose is to induce a brief stressful state. The reason for consciously generated bouts of acute stress is to train your mind and body how to downregulate your system when the body is approaching or entered a fight-or-flight response. Stressors, including such things as exercise, cold water swimming or ice baths, sauna, and intermittent fasting, create an opportunity for healthy adaptations if adequate downregulation recovery happens. So, stress is not inherently bad—but chronic stress is.

One such example of a stressful breathing practice is the Wim Hof method, where the practitioner consciously hyperventilates by taking 30 to 50 forceful and rapid breaths.* The immediate sensations include tingling, cold hands and feet, and lightness of head, and sometimes altered states of consciousness, all of which are classic symptoms of hyperventilation because of disturbance to blood gases. In the Wim Hof method, right after the hyperventilating breathing that sends the sympathetic nervous system into overdrive, the practitioner deescalates by holding their breath after an exhale and consciously slows their heartbeat. Essentially what is happening is the practitioner is actively stressing the body, and they then apply relaxation techniques. Research is ongoing as to the efficacy of the Wim Hof method and there is anecdotal evidence of beneficial mental health adaptations, increased resilience, and ability to manage pain.[2,†] Nevertheless, there is long-standing medical evidence that demonstrates a host of potential adverse effects to hyperventilating, including increased risk of cardiac arrhythmia, epileptic seizures, tinnitus, cramps, and spasms.[3]

There are other popular hyperventilation breathing practices such as rebirthing and holotropic breathwork that

---

* It should be noted that the Wim Hof method (WHM) of breathing is not tummö-style breathing, as many popular writers and commentators, including James Nestor and Dr. Andrew Huberman, have written and often stated. Wim Hof has stated that he never learned tummö and only read about the practice from 19th-century spiritual adventurers like Lama Anagarika Govinda and Alexandra David-Néel. Breathing during tummö is not fast nor powerful like in the WHM, but rather very slow. And the breath-holding techniques are completely different in tummö than in the WHM. In the WHM, the extended breath hold is on the exhale. During tummö, the breath hold is after the inhale and includes a "swallowing of the breath" and then active intra-abdominal pressure with a pulling up on the perineum and downward pressure from the throat area, known as *bandhas*. In tummö, the belly bulges out during the breath hold, which is why it is known as "vase breathing." Bandhas are essential in tummö, as in pranayama, and are not taught in WHM.

† Patrick McKeown and Anastasis Tzanis explore the physiological and psychological impacts of the Wim Hof method and the risks involved with voluntary hyperventilation in *Breathing for Yoga: Applying the Science Behind Ancient Wisdom In a Modern World*. They both offer serious words of caution.

are used therapeutically to process trauma and release emotions. Both rebirthing and holotropic breathing involve rhythmic, powerful breathing that turns on the sympathetic response, in part, by decreasing oxygen delivery to the brain, like in the Wim Hof method. Though useful in certain situations and with appropriate safety measures, and always with a trained guide or therapist, such stress-inducing breathing techniques should be approached with caution.

While some of the exercises and practices in this book will dial up your sympathetic nervous system, none are intended to move you into a hyperventilated state.

If hyperventilation causes stress to the nervous system, the converse follows: when you are breathing lightly, you increase your parasympathetic response, that rest-and-digest mode. With light breathing, blood circulation increases, and there is a more efficient uptake of oxygen to your brain and tissues because your blood gases are balanced. Your respiratory rate decreases because your parasympathetic nervous system releases acetylcholine, a neurotransmitter that causes muscles to relax and promotes memory.[‡] Breathing lightly through the nose is the preferred way to recover your breath when you become breathless, whether after high-intensity exercise, from physical exertion like carrying heavy bags of groceries into your house, or from fright. We'll discuss specific ways to recover your breath in Part II.

Though it may seem counterintuitive, you're able to take larger, more satisfying breaths when you breathe lightly and slowly through the nose. To demonstrate this point, try an experiment with the following two types of

---

‡   Acetylcholine is the chief neurotransmitter of the parasympathetic nervous system that contracts smooth muscles, dilates blood vessels, increases bodily secretions, and slows heart rate.

breaths to compare: first a powerful breath pattern and then a light breath pattern.

POWERFUL BREATH PATTERN

- Sit down—don't do this standing. First, notice your breathing.

- Take a few normal breaths and then progressively increase the strength.

- Inhale and exhale very powerfully 10 to 15 times through the nose or mouth.

- Then let go of the powerful breath pattern.

- Notice what is happening in your body and mind.

- Notice if your heart rate increased. Notice if there is tingling or heat felt in your hands or face. Is there ringing in your ears? What else do you notice? How did that make you feel?

- You've just turned up your sympathetic nervous system with those 10 to 15 breaths.

  Next, try this:

LIGHT BREATH PATTERN

- Sit down.

- Take a few normal breaths.

- Then, start inhaling and exhaling very lightly through your nose. Try not to move the hairs inside your nose as you breathe.

- Breathe lightly and slow, being patient. Observe the movement of air through your nostrils. Notice how the air feels cool inside the nasal cavity.

- If you must breathe through the mouth, be attentive to the feeling in the back of the throat. Very light inhalations.

- Exhale lightly as well. No need to force anything. Feel the warm air moving out of your body.

- After 10 to 15 breaths, let go of the light breathing.

- Notice what happened in your body and mind. How do you feel? What physical sensations are most prominent?

- Did your heart rate slow down? Perhaps sweet salvia formed in your mouth. Maybe you even yawned?

- You've just dialed up your parasympathetic nervous system with those 10 to 15 light breaths.

The Second Dial: Pace of Your Breath—Slow to Quick

The pace of your breath, also known as respiratory rate, is perhaps the most accessible dial with which you can adjust your nervous system. A fast-paced breath turns the dial up on your sympathetic dominance, while a slow-paced breath moves you toward a parasympathetic response. Breathe quick and you feel increasing energy; breathe slowly and you feel relaxation.

Like the strength of the breath (the first dial), there is a time and place for different paces of breathing. Healthy adults take 8 to 16 breaths per minute when at rest. When you meditate or employ specific slow-breathing techniques, like the one you will learn below, you may breathe four to six breaths per minute or slower, which usually induces the relaxation response. Studies have shown that the recitation of the Ave Maria (Hail Mary) rosary or specific yoga mantras slowed respiration to almost exactly six breaths per minute that evidenced enhanced heart rate variability, which is a common marker of cardiovascular strength.[4]

In my yogic breath training in India, we practiced super-slow nasal breathing at the rate of one breath per minute—a 20-second inhale and a 40-second exhale—for a quarter hour or longer prior to meditation. While that might be an extreme example, it shows that with a small amount of training, we can gain acute control over our respiratory rate.[5]

When you are jogging or dancing or doing other forms of exercise where the metabolic demand is high, it is normal for your breathing pace to increase to 40 to 60 breaths per minute, or even higher if you're cycling up a steep hill or swimming as fast as you can. The reason for taking more breaths is because your body is consuming more oxygen and producing more carbon dioxide, which needs to be expelled by exhaling. When the physical demand is not as intense, it is ideal to consciously slow the pace of your breath down—we'll discuss specific ways to do this in Chapter 10.

Sometimes your breathing rate increases because of psychological stress, such as right before speaking publicly, the thought of a tenuous financial predicament, or because a past traumatic episode has been stirred. If you can recognize through interoceptive awareness when your sympathetic nervous system is increasing and employ slow breathing, this will allow you to gain some control over your response. Remember AIR—awareness, intervention, regulation. You can slow your heart rate down by extending your exhalation, so the longer you spend on the outbreath, the more your nervous system relaxes.

To set a consistent pace of breathing, you can use specific cadences of inhales and exhales, like an inner metronome. The benefit of using a cadence is that you can precisely turn the breathing dial on your nervous system in the direction you want. If you breathe in for longer than you breathe out, you turn up the dial on your sympathetic nervous system. If you exhale for a longer duration than you inhale, this is usually relaxing. Imagine a grief-stricken person wailing. We can see them inhaling for about twice as long as they are exhaling. Or if somebody is frightened and trying to escape a situation, they might be panting in a similar fashion. These are two examples of the sympathetic nervous system–induced fight-or-flight breathing.

Let's look at individuals who have mastered Cadence Breathing, such as Olympic biathletes who combine cross-country skiing and target shooting. The skiing portion is extremely intense physically, sending their heart rates to nearly their maximums. The target shooting portion requires them to switch physiological gears within seconds, slowing their breath, heart rate, and thoughts so their body and rifle are as motionless as possible. It is as if you run as hard as you can up a long flight of stairs and then try to thread a needle.

When the biathlete is approaching the target and their heart rate is extremely high, how do they consciously intervene as they are lying down and taking aim at their target? They need to switch quickly from an overstimulated nervous system to one that can calmly perform a focused task. They use the same tools you are using in your breathing tool kit—using interoceptive awareness and attuning the dials on the nervous system. The athlete gathers their attention on their breath and consciously lengthens the exhalation, relaxing the face, jaw, and torso. Their intero-ceptive awareness feels the slowing of the heart rate, and they continue to extend their exhale, which allows for a relaxed focus in concentration, and in between heart-beats when their body and rifle is stillest, *bang!* they pull the trigger.

We do not need the breathing precision of an Olympic biathlete. But we do need to be able to slow our breathing pace down if we want to breathe how we want to feel.

Think of a time when you've been provoked by your child or sibling and your heart rate spiked, but it would be best not to react in that overstimulated state. Maybe you step on your child's LEGOs, or your brother or sister provokes you during a holiday family dinner. Or, maybe at home there is a medical emergency for a family member. In situations like these, the best course of action is not to react habitually in an overstimulated and cognitively clouded state.

So, what to do? Initiate a breathing intervention by immediately extending your exhalation—this single respi-ratory act creates the conditions for you to make better decisions. The same goes for those times when our stress, anger, anxiety, and other charged emotional states might impair our appropriate response. When you breathe out for longer than you breathe in, your rest-and-relax mode is turned on—know this and use it to your benefit.

Next, we will practice 4:6 Cadence Breathing, a pattern that induces a parasympathetic nervous system response. This cadence aligns heart rate oscillations with breathing, creating resonance frequency, commonly known as the flow state.

PRACTICE

4:6 Cadence Breathing

You'll inhale for a 4 count and exhale for a 6 count. Counting is done silently in the mind. There is no breath holding, but allow the natural pause to happen at the top and bottom of the breath. Inhale to about 70 percent capacity, and exhale slowly.

- Find a comfortable position, seated or lying down.

- Briefly think: *With this Cadence Breathing, may I calm my body and mind.*

- Notice how your body feels, and notice what is happening in your mind.

- Turn your attention to your breath for a moment and practice breath awareness. No need to change anything. Just notice the breath.

- Breathe in and out of your nose.

- Place one hand over your navel and notice the movement as you breathe.

- Now, begin your 4:6 Cadence Breathing.

- Inhale slowly for a count of 4.

- Let the breath at the top naturally pause for a moment.

- Exhale slowly out the nose for a count of 6.

- Allow the breath to pause naturally for a moment at the bottom of the exhale.

- And continue for two to three minutes.

- You may notice after a minute or so that you can feel your heart rate increase on the inhalation and slow down during the exhale. This is a common interoceptive insight during Cadence Breathing.

- If your mind wanders off the breath or you lose count, don't worry. That's normal. When you recognize you've been distracted, simply come back to feeling your hand on your belly and the movement of the inhale and exhale and continue with the 4:6 cadence.

- At the conclusion, let go of the breathing intervention and notice for a minute or so how your body and mind feel.

The Third Dial: Depth of Your Breath—Shallow to Deep

We have just covered two breathing dials on our nervous system—breathing strength (lightly to powerfully) and breathing pace (slowly to quickly). The final dial you can adjust is the depth of the breath, which controls the total volume of air you bring in on each breath.[§]

When we are upset, we've all been told sometimes by a well-meaning friend to "take a deep breath." The suggestion our friend makes is because taking a big breath is meant to calm our agitation. But, if you watch yourself or others perform that "big, deep breath," what do you observe?

Do we fill the lungs gradually and fully, dialing down our nervous system? After we inhale, is there a slow exhale that tells the brain it is okay to rest and digest? Do we see

---

[§]   This is sometimes referred to as *tidal volume*, which is the amount of air that moves in or out of the lungs with each respiratory cycle. It measures around 500 mL in an average healthy adult male and approximately 400 mL in a healthy female. It is a vital clinical parameter that allows for proper ventilation to take place.

the face relax, as if stress is draining away with the one "deep breath"?

Or, on the other hand, do you observe that "deep breath" taken with kind of gasping into a mouth that's wide open? Maybe the breath is taken so powerfully through the nose that the sides of the nose collapse from the suction. Do the shoulders lift? And was there tension in the face?

If you were to conduct your own "take a deep breath experiment" on your friends and family, I suspect the majority of those you observe won't take that deep breath in a light, slow, and full manner. Rather, they may put a strong, sharp gasp of an inhale, tensing their face and jaw, breathing quickly through the mouth. Their chest likely puffs outward, and their neck muscles might even tighten. If this was the case, the breath was not "deep" but rather was quite shallow and unsatisfying. And the volume of air they bring in is much less than if they breathed in slowly and through the nose. Their brain senses this quick shallow breath and registers a threat is present, as if a grizzly bear just knocked down the front door. What does it look and sound like when someone is startled with fear? Are their mouths and eyes wide open, and are they gasping? This is likely not the way you or your friends and family want to feel upon the suggested "just take a deep breath."

The hallmark of a deep breath is that it is driven by your primary breathing muscles—the diaphragm and intercostals. Your dome-shaped diaphragm muscle separates the thoracic cavity from the abdominal cavity. The intercostals are the muscles in between your individual ribs. You can feel your diaphragm with your fingertips.

Try this right now as you are reading or listening to this book; put your fingers on your sternum and move them down, prodding inward around and below the edge of your ribs. Push in and under—use both hands. It may feel tender, so be gentle. This is where your diaphragm attaches to the rib cage. Let your fingers roll slightly under your ribs, moving slowly. Keep breathing and feel the changing pressure. With your fingers slightly curled under your ribs, take a slow, deep breath to fill up your lungs, and you'll feel your diaphragm move as your rib cage expands and then contracts. I highly recommend doing this diaphragmatic self-massage daily with your fingers or a massage ball, roller, or slightly deflated volleyball.

Diaphragmatic Breathing

Like the rest of your respiratory system, the diaphragm functions automatically, but you can also take control over it for specific breathing interventions. The automation is conducted from the brain stem, the most ancient part of your brain at the base of the skull. Every breath is taken with a signal that fires from the brain to the diaphragm via nerves. When you inhale, the diaphragm contracts and flattens out, decreasing the intrathoracic pressure, which draws air into the lungs like the pulling up of a syringe. Your ribs expand outward and slightly lift as your lungs inflate. The contracting movement of the diaphragm and expansion of the lungs causes downward pressure on the abdominal area.

Diaphragmatic breathing creates an invigorating up-and-down motion that massages and stimulates your heart, liver, stomach, and large intestines. Even the kidneys, located at the back of your torso, directly benefit from the rhythmic motion of the diaphragm. As the diaphragm descends, the organs underneath are gently pushed forward, backward, and sideways. This expansion of the abdomen gives the impression of breathing into the stomach, even though there is no respiration occurring in the belly. This is why diaphragmatic breathing is sometimes called "Belly Breathing."

During your exhalation, the diaphragm relaxes and returns to its dome shape, thereby creating higher intrathoracic pressure that forces air out of your lungs. This cycle of contraction and relaxation of the diaphragm is essential for proper respiration.

When you breathe diaphragmatically, it is important to feel yourself expanding in all directions—forward, to the sides, and backward—rather than just vertically. Recall the "deep breath experiment" from earlier—many people you'll observe raise their shoulders when they take a deep breath. Here, I'm encouraging you to explore breathing outward rather than upward. When you inhale slowly, feel the pressure and allow your ribs to expand horizontally, rather than immediately breathing into your upper chest. Continue to expand in 360 degrees. In the Buteyko method and Oxygen Advantage system, a belt is worn around the midsection, not unlike the cotton belt I wore around my lower ribs when I was first studying pranayama, to provide gentle resistance to train in diaphragmatic breathing.

Let's practice diaphragmatic breathing—or if you want to call it Belly Breathing, that is also totally fine!

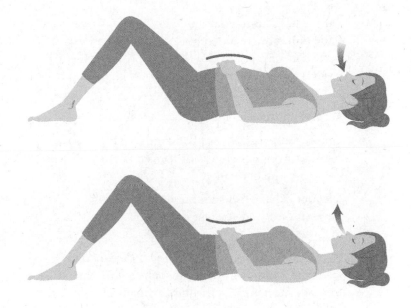

PRACTICE

Diaphragmatic Breathing

- Find a comfortable position, seated or lying down.
- Place one hand on your sternum and the other on your belly.
- Think to yourself: *May my diaphragmatic breathing bring me strength so I can be of service to others.*
- Turn your attention to your breath for a moment and practice breath awareness. No need to change; just notice how you are breathing this moment.
- Breathe lightly in and out of your nose.

- Shift your focus to your hands and notice which hand or hands are moving. No need to breathe a particular way, just notice for a few breaths which hand is moving on the inhale and which hand is moving on the exhale.

- Let's begin to breathe diaphragmatically.

- On your inhale, feel your hand on your belly move outward. Try not to have any movement in your chest. Breathe normally.

- On your exhale, feel your hand on your belly move inward, and you can gently press in for a bit of feedback.

- Continue to feel your belly expand on the inhale. Don't push your belly out; rather allow it to expand from the movement of the breath and diaphragm.

- On the exhale, the belly moves inward naturally.

- Continue for 5 to 10 breaths.

- Now, change your hand position so that your thumbs are touching your floating ribs on your sides.

- On your inhale, notice your belly moving outward and feel your ribs expanding.

- On your exhale, notice your belly moving inward and feel your ribs contracting.

- Continue for 5 to 10 breaths.

- At the conclusion, let go of the breathing intervention and notice for a minute how your body and mind feel.

I encourage you to play with your three breathing dials to adjust your nervous system. Adjust the strength of your breath from light to powerful and see what happens to your mental focus and energy. Change the pace of your breath from quick to slow when you are lightly exercising and observe the effect. And when you are meditating or having a quiet cup of tea, try breathing diaphragmatically and feel yourself expand horizontally rather than vertically. If the words *Belly Breathing* remind you to feel your inhalation expand around the navel area, go with that. When you gain experiential understanding of how and when to adjust these dials, the ability to breathe how you want to feel is within your grasp.

KEY INSIGHTS

- Attune your nervous system by consciously adjusting the strength, pace, and depth of your breathing. Using these breathing dials is the second tool in your breathing tool kit.

- Lengthening your exhale, breathing out for longer than you breathe in, is a reliable way to self-regulate. Practice extended exhales and become adept at this simple method so you can apply it in the moment to acute stressors.

- For a satisfying and nourishing deep breath, rather than quick and forceful inhale, take air in slowly and lightly through the nose, filling from the bottom up. As you breathe in, feel yourself expand not only vertically but also laterally.

Chapter 4

BREATHING THROUGH YOUR NOSE

There are many actionable practices in this book. But the single most important habit to take away from these pages is to breathe through your nose, day and night. Awareness is necessary, and breathing interventions immediately impact your nervous system. But it is habitual nasal breathing—rather than mouth breathing—that will contribute to the long-term benefits to your mental and physical health. As James Nestor wrote in *Breath*, "The nose is the silent warrior; the gatekeeper of our bodies, pharmacist to our minds, and weather vane to our emotions."[1]

You can start right now—as you continue reading or listening to this book, gently close your lips with your teeth not touching, rest your tongue on your upper palate, and breathe lightly through your nose. It might feel a bit forced at first, but nose breathing is a habit and a habit must be established before it can be improved. Moving into the rest of the day, remind yourself to nasal breathe with the simple mantra of this book: *Keep it nasal.*

When walking to and from your house today—*keep it nasal.*

When you are on your computer or scrolling on your phone—*keep it nasal.*

When you are in the kitchen preparing a meal—*keep it nasal.*

When you are lying down to sleep—*keep it nasal.*

In nearly all situations, except when you are speaking, eating, or exercising intensely—*keep it nasal.*

Nose Breathing	Mouth Breathing
• Serene mind	• Restless mind
• Restful sleep	• Disrupted sleep
• Refreshed awakening	• Fatigued mornings
• Sustained energy	• Daytime lethargy
• Clarity of thought	• Mental fog
• Relaxed focus	• Scattered
• Heightened concentration	• Distracted

The human respiratory system evolved with its primary tool being the nose, not the mouth. The mouth developed to support digestion and facilitate communication but is far inferior to the nose when it comes to optimizing respiration. Your nose is designed for breathing, and your mouth is designed for eating. Before we look at why nasal breathing is far more beneficial than breathing through the mouth, let's be clear about what exactly "mouth breathing" is.

Nasal Breathing vs. Mouth Breathing

Mouth breathing is breathing in and out through the mouth for sustained periods of time and at regular intervals while awake or asleep. Mouth breathing is often shallow, similar to panting. It is sometimes audible and often involves the up and down movement of the shoulders and chest area. Mouth breathers tend to sigh often. Mouth breathers take in too much air, disrupting the optimal balance of their blood gases, namely oxygen and carbon dioxide. The effect of chronic mouth breathing is hyperventilation, which causes brain fog, belching and bloating, dry mouth and cracked lips, cold hands and feet, and easily becoming breathless. And, mouth breathing exposes the lungs more readily than nasal breathing to everything in the environment, from pollutants to mold.

As mentioned earlier, the only times breathing through your mouth is necessary is when the metabolic demands increase, such as:

- When you are in dangerous or threatening situation, like when you are being chased

- When exercising at an intense effort, for example, with short and high-intensity bursts of effort, or while swimming

- When there is a blockage in your nasal area from injury or illness

Otherwise, mouth breathing is your back-up ventilation system to nasal breathing.

Benefits of Nasal Breathing

When you breathe, air is drawn into your lungs—and the route that air flows in, either through the mouth or nose, matters.

When you breathe through the mouth, the air passes quickly and directly into the lungs, only passing over the teeth and tonsils before descending the windpipe into the lungs. It is very difficult to maintain diaphragmatic breathing through the mouth for any length of time. Instead, mouth breathing encourages inefficient upper-chest breathing, which causes a sympathetic nervous system response, signaling to the brain that you're in a stressful situation.

Nose breathing, on the other hand, engages the diaphragm and encourages slower breathing that cues your relaxation response. More significantly, however, is that nasal breathing optimizes oxygenation delivery to your brain and organs by as much as 18 percent over mouth breathing![2] How does this happen through the nose?

When you breathe through your nose, the air enters the nostrils into an extensive network of channels, pockets, and canals formed by boney turbinates. This mazelike area of the paranasal sinuses inside your skull has the volume of your fist and is lined with cilia, tiny hair follicles that filter the air of toxins. You have as many hair follicles inside your sinuses as you do on your head. There is also a layer of beneficial mucus that covers the paranasal area. When you inhale harmful bacteria into your nasal area, this layer of mucus secretes antimicrobial proteins, protecting against the agent before it moves into the lungs. Taken together, the cilia and mucus form an effective trapping system of inhaled pathogens and help to kill the bacteria, not letting them enter your lungs.[3]

Nose breathing protects you from inhaled pathogens, and the paranasal sinuses and turbinates form an elaborate air-conditioning system that spins, warms, and humidifies the air. This system cleanses and moistens the air before it reaches the tissues in your lungs, which have minimal defense on their own. In addition to all the benefits of purifying and conditioning the air, there are baroreceptors in your nasal area that help communicate to the brain to slow down your heart rate and blood pressure.

None of this protection or air-conditioning happens when you breathe through your mouth. In fact, there are myriad downsides to mouth breathing, including facial deformities beginning in childhood, bad breath, poor sinus drainage due to lack of filtration, sleep disruption and apnea, gum and periodontal disease, postural problems, dehydration, and increased anxiety and panic attacks, to name just a handful. In Part II, we will discuss corrective measures for persistent mouth breathers.¶

Harnessing the Power of Nitric Oxide

Another benefit of nasal breathing is that it harnesses the molecule nitric oxide. The molecules of nitric oxide offer potent protection against airborne viruses, bacteria, and allergens.[4] Nitric oxide forms in the lining of the nasal airways and during nasal inhalation is distributed throughout your airway and lungs. Nitric oxide is a powerful vasodilator that opens airways and improves respiratory function. This reduces inflammation in and around the airways, making it easier for us to breathe. Furthermore, nitric oxide diminishes oxidative stress associated with pollution, exercise, and other environmental factors.

¶   It is important to note that some of us have serious structural challenges with our nose and sinuses, such as deviated septums, collapsed nostrils, or chronically inflamed turbinates. This can make nasal breathing almost impossible. In these cases, please see your ear, nose, and throat physician.

None of the benefits of nitric oxide offers happen if you inhale through your mouth.

Let's do a brief exercise to experience the nitric oxide that is present in your nasal passageway. This exercise will open your nostrils, decongest your sinuses, and open your lungs.

You begin by exhaling and holding your breath for a short period. While you are holding your breath, nitric oxide is pooling in your sinuses. After holding your breath for 5 to 30 seconds, inhale slowly through the nose to distribute the amazing vasodilating molecules throughout your sinuses and bronchial pathways. Let's give it a try.

PRACTICE

Opening Your Nasal Breathing with Nitric Oxide

- Assume a comfortable seated position. Lightly close your lips.

- Breathe normally through the nose.

- Notice if there is any congestion or constriction when you breathe.

- Notice if one nostril is more open than the other.

- After a few normal breaths, exhale and lightly pinch your nose and hold your breath, keeping your mouth closed.

- Gently nod your head or move your torso back and forth until you feel a relatively strong urge to breathe (5 to 30 seconds).

- Let go of your nose and gently breathe in through the nose, keeping your mouth closed.

- You are breathing in the nitric oxide that has been pooling in your nasal passageway.

- When you breathe in, avoid taking a quick, sharp breath. Rather, calmly and slowly breathe through your nose.

- Repeat 4 to 5 times, or until you feel the nasal passageway is unblocked.

Nasal Breathing and the Vagus Nerve

Another benefit of nasal breathing is the role it plays in stimulating your vagus nerve. The vagus nerve is the main nerve of your parasympathetic nervous system. The vagus nerve attaches to the base of the brain and travels down the neck, through the heart, lungs, diaphragm, and stomach. Because it is a meandering system, the vagus nerve takes its name from the Latin word meaning "wandering." It's a two-way communication system, but most of the information that moves through the vagus nerve are signals from the body being relayed to the brain. For example, when you breathe slowly, the brain receives signals from the vagus nerve that you are safe, that you don't have to stress about your immediate situation. As you experienced earlier during the 4:6 Cadence Breathing when you exhaled slowly, your heart rate and blood pressure decreased, and this too is information sent by your vagus nerve to your brain that you can relax. Slow breathing is one of the quickest and most efficient ways to stimulate the vagus nerve and reduce stress in the body and mind.[5]

The health of your vagus nerve is measured by vagal tone, a term coined by Stephen Porges in his polyvagal theory, which is the ability for your parasympathetic nervous system to activate and adapt in response to stressful challenges. Breathing interventions that stimulate the vagus nerve regulate our internal bodily processes, such as glucose levels and inflammation, more efficiently. Mentally, we're better able to regulate our attention and emotions, especially our response to acute and chronic stress. And socially, with a higher vagal tone, we're more skilled in navigating interpersonal interactions and in forging positive connections with those around us. [6],**

Because the vagus nerve passes through so many parts of the body, there are other ways to enhance your vagal tone other than slow breathing, such as:[7]

- Gargling
- Meditation
- Singing and chanting
- Laughter and social connection
- Cold water immersion
- Sexual intimacy
- Yoga, tai chi, and exercise
- Humming

The Benefits of Humming

Humming is particularly effective at increasing your vagal tone. Humming? Yes, just good ol' fashioned humming along to your favorite song, be it to Beethoven's "Ode to Joy," a hip-hop song, or chanting of OM.

** Vagal tone is measured using a metric called heart rate variability (HRV). The heart doesn't beat like a metronome, but instead its speed is a response to the current circumstances inside and outside the body. The constant fluctuations in heart rate are called HRV, which is measured as the time and frequency between heart beats. The more variability there is between these beats, the more adaptable your system is, in particular your resiliency to stress.

Humming elongates your exhale because there is resistance to the air that is exhaled. This resistance is caused by your vocal cords closing slightly, which creates the humming sound. You know that an extended exhale creates a parasympathetic response, increasing your vagal tone and relaxing your body and mind.

Secondly, the vibration of the humming stimulates the vagus nerve that runs in the inner canal of your ear. Research indicates that this vibration deactivates parts of the brain, principally the amygdala, which is associated with depression as well as your fight-or-flight response.[8] The magical frequency to hum seems to be right around 120 Hertz, which is in the key of B.

And thirdly, when you hum at a low pitch and strongly (no need to be shy!) you greatly increase the amount of nitric oxide pooling in your nasal passage. Separate studies have evidenced a 15-fold increase in nitric oxide production when compared to quiet nasal exhalation.[9] The studies were conducted on people who suffered from chronic rhinosinusitis and allergies. After humming four times a day for around five minutes, for four days, their "chronic rhinosinusitis was essentially eliminated," and they breathed for the first time in years with clear sinuses. The primary reasons for the results were attributed to elevated levels of nitric oxide and its associated antifungal agency.[10]

I was introduced to humming practice during my pranayama training in Nepal and India and specifically when we studied the 15th-century text *Hatha Yoga Pradipika*. In the text, there are eight different pranayama practices taught, and one of them is called *bhramari*, which means "bee" in Sanskrit. This practice is given that name because the hummed *mmmm* sound mimics the sound of a buzzing bee. Bhramari is a very uncomplicated pranayama practice as there is no breath holding, specific counting or ratio, or specified bodily posture. I was taught to block my ears with my thumbs and place my middle and ring fingers gently over my eyes. This helps to immerse yourself in the feeling and vibration, but it is not absolutely necessary—the main benefits come from the humming vibration. Inhaling slowly, I'd exhale with the long humming, directing the low hum between my eyebrows.

Bhramari is part of a collection of practices where the senses are withdrawn from the outside world and redirected inward toward the source of experience, the interoception we spoke about earlier. [11] The promise of bhramari, according to my teacher, was the release of physical tension in the upper part of the body, soothing of mental tension, and balancing of the energies within the subtle energy body. He also mentioned that daily practice of the bee humming practice eventually leads the yogi to the psychic landscape of the third eye (ajna chakra), where beatific visions and spiritual realizations unfold. Sometimes we hummed as a group indoors for an hour, and the harmonics created among the group, even with my ears closed, seemed to enter my body with sonic energy from all directions.

Practice humming spontaneously as you go about your day, or it can be a more formal practice session like the one below. If you are congested, practice the nasal unblocking practice for a few minutes to open your sinuses.

PRACTICE

Bhramari Pranayama—Humming Bee

- Assume a comfortable position, seated or lying down, or you can practice walking.

- Briefly think: *May my humming practice calm my nervous system so I find deeper connections with others.*

- Turn your attention to your breath for a moment and practice breath awareness. No need to change, just notice how you are breathing this moment.

- Breathe slowly in and out of your nose.

- Now, turn your attention within and notice how you feel. Just notice.

- Gently close your eyes.

- Relax your jaw and face. Keep your teeth slightly parted, with your lips sealed. Place your tongue on the roof of your mouth.

- Then, inhale fully through the nostrils.

- Lightly plug your ears with your thumbs and cover your eyes with your fingers.

- As you exhale, make the sound *mmmm* like the buzzing sound of a bumble bee.

- Make the hum low in pitch. Don't be shy about the volume, but no need to force the exhalation and hum.

- Relax and extend your humming sound.

- Listen and feel inside of the skull as you hum.

- Direct the energetic vibration to the center of the skull, behind your eyebrows, rather than to your chest or elsewhere.

- Inhale and repeat the humming on the exhalation.

- Continue for 15 to 20 rounds or for as long as you like.

- At the conclusion of your humming, let your hands rest in your lap. Remain silent for a few minutes. Feel the sensations inside the skull. If the mind begins to analyze the sensations or wanders into thinking, gently come back to the feeling.

- Finally, let go of the breathing intervention and notice for a minute or so how your body and mind feel.

Nasal Breathing and Sleep

I expressed above my hope that you breathe through your nose (almost) all the time, and that means while you sleep. If you live to be 80 years old, you'll spend about 26 years sleeping. Yes, you'll be asleep about a third of your life. And, if you add how much time you spend *trying* to fall asleep, bump up that number to 33 years in bed.

If you spend your sleeping hours with your mouth closed, you'll have better rest and improved cognitive functions when you wake up, and all your major organs will benefit. Nasal breathing while sleeping is a critical and sometimes little-mentioned element to sound sleep hygiene.

Sleep hygiene is a habit adopted for optimal sleep and includes both the environment and your behavior. An important factor to good sleep hygiene is having a consistent sleep routine. This means going to bed and getting up at the same time every day, even on the weekends, so that your body's internal clock (circadian rhythm) is consistent. When you go to bed and wake up at the same time each day, this reinforces your body's natural inclination for sound, restful sleep. To help set that circadian rhythm, spend 10 minutes outside to receive light into your eyes within a half-hour upon waking and another 10 minutes around dusk. Included in healthy sleep hygiene is avoiding caffeine and alcohol late in the evening, avoiding screens for at least a couple hours before bed, not eating food for a few hours before sleep, and establishing a calming night-time routine that helps you relax.

With that said, you may have the perfect sleep hygiene, but if you are spending your sleeping hours with your mouth open, you won't be able to extract the restorative benefits from sleep. All the advantages of nasal breathing we discussed earlier—from filtering, warming, and humidi-fying the air as well as maintaining increasing oxygenation of your brain and tissue, including your sex organs—apply to when you are sleeping. None of that happens if you are a mouth breather during sleep. Additionally, breathing through your mouth while you sleep is unhealthy because it leads to sleep disruptions like snoring and sleep apnea, both of which are linked to poor cardiovascular health, depression, and sexual dysfunction. Snoring is a clear sign of mouth breathing.

How you breathe during your day-to-day life impacts how you breathe during sleep and vice versa. Extensive research shows that adults who mouth breathe during sleep are more likely to experience breathing disordered sleep, fatigue, decreased productivity, and poorer quality of life than those who breathe through their nose.[12] As we get older, mouth breathing often becomes more prev-alent. From the age 40, you're 60 percent more likely to spend at least half the night breathing through an open mouth. And in postmenopausal women, the risk of sleep apnea increases by 200 percent.[13] It's important to recog-nize that snoring and sleep apnea aren't exclusively caused by mouth breathing; additional factors such as metabolic concerns, excess adipose tissue, and anatomical character-istics also play a role.

Research is also clear that mouth breathing puts you more at risk for dental problems, including cavities. In children, the harmful effects of mouth breathing during the day and night are far greater, since it is during these formative years that breathing shapes the orofacial structures, including their palate. Not treating a mouth-breathing habit in children for extended periods of time can set the stage for lifelong respiratory problems and cognitive challenges.

There are a number of reasons why the mouth opens during sleep that include:

- Nasal congestion: If you have a cold or allergies, you may breathe through your mouth to compensate for the blocked nasal passages. The nasal opening practice on page 56 helps to open your sinuses before bed.

- Sleep apnea: "Apnea" means to stop, and sleep apnea is a disorder in which your airway becomes blocked while sleeping, causing you to stop breathing and then gasp through the mouth to begin breathing again. It is a very serious health issue about which you should consult with your doctor.

- Habitual mouth breathing: If you habitually breathe through your mouth during the day, you will likely continue to do so while sleeping.

- Jaw or tongue position: The position of your jaw and tongue can cause your mouth to open during sleep. For example, if the tongue falls back into the throat, this can cause the mouth to open.

Without a personalized sleep study, which is usually done overnight in a laboratory, how do you know if you're mouth breathing at night? There are home sleep tests where you wear a monitor that collects bio data. Often, your spouse or partner tells you that you are wheezing, snoring, or gasping. Or, if you wake up with a dry mouth, cracked lips, or tiredness that lingers into the late morning, these are signs you are probably mouth breathing.

Additionally, if you need to urinate multiple times during the night, this is a likely sign that you are mouth breathing. The reason is because mouth breathing disrupts deep sleep. During deep sleep, many hormones are released, including vasopressin, which regulates water balance in the body. Our vasopressin levels rise during deep sleep, reducing the need to urinate. If our sleep is disrupted, however, vasopressin levels drop, kidneys release water, and we not only need to urinate but also feel thirsty.

Mouth Taping

How, then, can we sleep with our mouth closed? The answer to this question is simple but may surprise you. You need to tape your mouth closed. There is no other more passive way to create immediate improvements to your sleep quality and overall health than placing a stamp-size strip of medical tape on your lips. The aim of using mouth tape isn't to forcibly seal your lips, but rather to serve as a gentle reminder for your muscles to relax. I said earlier that the single most important takeaway from this book is to breathe habitually through your nose nearly all the time, and mouth taping is a necessary practice for nearly everyone, especially if you are suffering from snoring, chronic sleep apnea, or asthma.

Here are nine reasons to begin mouth taping:

1. Improves nasal breathing
2. Increases sleep quality
3. Reduces snoring
4. Reduces risk of sleep apnea
5. Reduce risk of dry mouth and bad breath
6. Increase oxygen uptake
7. Promotes diaphragmatic breathing
8. Reduce stress and anxiety during sleep
9. Improves dental health

Not everyone needs to tape their mouth. If you sleep with your mouth closed all the time, it is not necessary. But it is hard to know if you always keep your mouth closed while sleeping. There is no harm in taping your mouth if you are already keeping your mouth closed. Mouth taping is a simple and effective solution and the payoff to your health and wellness is beyond measure.

PRACTICE

Sleeping with Your Mouth Closed

- Get yourself a roll of medical micropore grade, skin-safe tape (easily found at the pharmacy), or Myotape. Do not use household or athletic tape.

- Clear your nasal passage by lightly blowing your nose, using a neti pot, or using some other rinse.

- If you find your nasal passage closed, use the nasal opening practice on page 56.

- Tear off a piece of tape a bit larger than a stamp and place it over the center of your lips. The tape need not cover the entire mouth, only the middle of your lips, so you can still breathe out the sides on either side if needed. You can also use two strips, making an X over your lips or use Myotape that gently draws your lips together.

- Before turning off the lights, set your intention: *I'll sleep all night with my mouth closed.*

- Lie on your side and gently breathe through your nose as you fall asleep.

- In the morning, it is important to first moisten the tape with your tongue. Do not rip the tape off your lips—gently remove it after it has been moistened by your tongue or when you wash your face.

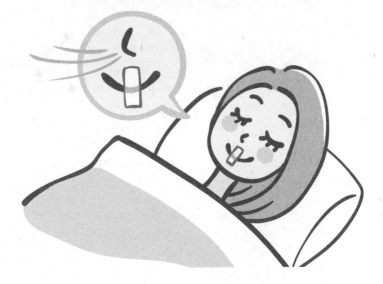

The medical tape used for this purpose is not strong enough to keep your mouth closed should you want to forcibly open your mouth. When people begin mouth taping, they often unknowingly take the tape off in the middle of the night. If this happens, just continue mouth taping until your facial and mouth muscles adapt.

Mouth taping is safe for nearly everyone (except for children younger than 5), though it should be avoided if you've been drinking excessive alcohol, have a vomit-related illness, or experience uncontrolled epilepsy.

If you have some hesitation or anxiety about mouth taping, try taping your mouth while on your computer or watching television to get a feel for it. Below is a suggested one-week schedule to get used to mouth taping.

PRACTICE

One Week to Get Used to Mouth Taping

- Apply a stamp-sized piece of micropore tape over your lips.

- Place the tongue on the upper palate and relax the face.

- When you want to remove the tape, do so by moistening it with your tongue and then pressing out with your tongue. Do not rip the tape off your lips.

Day 1: 10 minutes of mouth taping while seated and working on the computer or reading.

Day 2: 20 minutes of mouth taping while seated and working on the computer or reading or moving around the house.

Day 3: 1 hour of mouth taping seated or moving around the house.

Day 4: 1 hour of mouth taping around the house + 10 minutes while lying down before going to sleep.

Day 5: 1 hour of mouth taping around the house + 30 minutes before going to sleep.

Day 6: 2 hours of mouth taping around the house + 1 hour before going to sleep.

Day 7: 2 hours of mouth taping around the house + falling asleep with mouth taped.

KEY INSIGHTS

- Breathe through your nose (almost) all the time. Unless you are exercising intensely or have blocked sinuses, keep it nasal. Nasal breathing offers protection against pathogens and purifies and humidifies the air—none of which happen with mouth breathing. Nasal breathing is your third tool in your breathing tool kit.

- Harness the extraordinary benefits of nitric oxide with nasal breathing. Humming increases production of nitric oxide and stimulates your vagus nerve, the primary nerve for relaxation and digestion.

- Tape your mouth closed for improved sleep, to reduce or eliminate snoring, and to wake up restored physically and mentally.

Chapter 5

HOLDING YOUR BREATH

A normal cycle of breath has an inhale, a natural pause, then an exhale, and another pause, like a gentle wave ebbing and flowing. At any point along this rising and falling of the breath, you can take conscious control and suspend your breathing. You might fully inhale and hold your breath at the top, like we all used to do on the playground as kids or before we dove into the swimming pool. Or, you can fully exhale and hold your breath, like yogis do, pulling their belly button to their spine. It's possible to stairstep the breath in 25 percent and hold, take in another 25 percent and hold, and then inhale to full 100 percent capacity. You can stairstep out the exhale as well.

The average person without training can hold their breath after an inhale from 15 to 90 seconds, depending on various factors such as age, fitness level, and lung capacity. I have met masters of breathing in Tibet and India who hold their breath for well over 5 minutes while performing yogic postures. The most extreme example of breath holding has to be professional free divers who hold a single breath for over 20 minutes! You don't need to learn free divers' extreme methods to benefit from breath holding or even devote yourself to the austere life of a Himalayan yoga master. But learning how to consciously hold your breath for very short durations—just seconds at a time—can be a superpower for your emotional and physical well-being.

Before we learn why breath holding is a superpower, let's take a step back and consider what is the stimulation to breathe? And let's approach this experientially rather than just in theory.

- Wherever you are reading or listening to this book (except if you are driving), after your next exhale, suspend your breath; that is, hold your breath at the bottom of your exhale.

- Notice how you feel. Continue to hold. Try to hold your breath for longer than is comfortable.

- You probably feel some pressure in your torso, neck, or maybe your face.

- There may be a feeling of suspension or floating. Keep holding.

- After 15 to 20 seconds, there may be a feeling of the need to breathe. Relax but don't breathe.

- For some, it may be 30 to 40 seconds or longer. Finally, when there is a strong urge to breathe, notice the feeling and then inhale.

- Notice the feeling of relief.

- Within a second or two, you'll feel normal.

Why did you need to breathe after that period of breath holding? Many people will answer, "I needed air. I needed oxygen." That answer is incorrect, but that's okay. Most people make that assumption.

The reason you needed to breathe was not because you needed oxygen. In those 15 to 60 seconds, the oxygen saturation in your blood did not change—you had enough oxygen. The reason you felt the need to breathe was carbon dioxide was increasing in your system as you held your breath. This increase of carbon dioxide was sensed in the most ancient part of your brain that is responsible for basic survival. Your brain stem sends signals to your respiratory system to offload carbon dioxide by exhaling. Our stimulus to breathe is, in short, carbon dioxide.

To understand the relationship carbon dioxide has with oxygen when you breathe, we must venture for a moment to high school biology for a refresher on respiration.

Respiration 101

Respiration starts when you breathe in air. The air around you right now is about 78 percent nitrogen, 21 percent oxygen, and less than 1 percent other gases. As you inhale, you start the respiration process when the oxygen molecules that were just outside you now are in your lungs. This is truly a miracle that the air that you inhaled was hovering in the room around you just a few seconds ago and is already being used as energy in your body. Dr. Michael J. Stephens writes about the evolutionary development of the lungs in *Breath Taking: The Power, Fragility, and Future of Our Extraordinary Lungs* and beautifully observes, "The lungs are a mysterious and even mystical organ. They are our connection to the atmosphere, the organ that extracts the life force we need to exist."[1]

Every time you inhale, every few seconds, air travels down your trachea and branches into the bronchi of the right and left lungs and eventually expands the 600 million tiny balloon-like sacs called alveoli. Your alveoli look like tiny grapelike clusters and are made of capillaries that provide the exchange surface for oxygen to enter your bloodstream. In just one of your lungs, if the surface of all the alveoli was stretched out, an area about the size of a tennis court would be covered! After the oxygen molecules move into the lungs, through the alveoli and into your blood, they attach to a protein called hemoglobin. The hemoglobin is like a transport vehicle that delivers oxygen throughout your body. Your oxygen-rich blood flows through the heart, which pumps it into the arteries and capillaries and throughout your body, delivering the fuel for the cells in your brain, organs, and tissues.

As your cells use oxygen to produce energy for you to live, carbon dioxide and water are byproducts, which leave the cells and enter your bloodstream. In your biology class, the teacher probably called carbon dioxide a waste gas, but as we will see, it is anything but wasteful!

As carbon dioxide molecules move through the bloodstream, they pass through a cluster of cells in your aorta, carotid artery, and brain stem called chemoreceptors. These chemoreceptors are specialized sensors that detect changes in the chemical composition of your blood, particularly the levels of oxygen, carbon dioxide, and pH. This monitoring system provides a feedback loop to your respiratory centers in the brain stem. When carbon dioxide levels increase, like when you hold your breath or exercise, your brain and body tell you to exhale.

Let's pause for a moment—before completely exhaling—and go back within the body. It is very important that you understand that the impetus for the oxygen molecules to release from the hemoglobin and enter your cells (for energy) is the concentration of carbon dioxide in the blood. Think of hemoglobin as the vehicle, the four tires as oxygen molecules, and carbon dioxide as the pavement. Because carbon dioxide is acidic, it causes the four tires to fly off the vehicle, or in this case, the four oxygen molecules to release and enter the cells of your body. In other words, you bring in oxygen from outside, and the carbon dioxide that is within your body allows you to use that oxygen most efficiently. So, carbon dioxide is not a waste gas at all!

Your respiratory system tries to maintain homeostasis, which means balanced levels of oxygen, carbon dioxide, and pH in your blood. But when there is dysfunctional breathing, especially mouth breathing, that balance is lost because too much carbon dioxide is expelled from your body. With a lower concentration of carbon dioxide, what happens? We just said that carbon dioxide is what causes oxygen to be released into your brain and tissue. When you blow off too much carbon dioxide, oxygen stays bound to the hemoglobin in the blood and isn't delivered as readily. You feel lightheaded, weak, and faint because you have inefficient oxygen uptake into the cells. Conversely, when there are higher levels of carbon dioxide in the blood, more oxygen is delivered into your brain and organs more readily. The physiology is called the Bohr effect and was discovered in 1904 by the Danish physiologist Christian Bohr.[2] The Bohr effect describes how hemoglobin's oxygen-binding affinity is inversely related both to acidity and to the concentration of carbon dioxide.

Our brain represents only 2 percent of our total body weight but accounts for 20 percent of the oxygen consumption we breathe when we are at rest. So it's important that the oxygen arrives to the brain! The brain uses oxygen at a very rapid rate, and it's dependent on an uninterrupted supply for maintenance of its function and structural integrity. The brain doesn't have a large storage area for oxygen—it needs continuous replenishment of oxygen.

It follows that if you adapt your system to become less sensitive to carbon dioxide, when concentration levels rise in your blood, more oxygen is delivered to your cells. This physiological process is the reason short breath holds are a superpower because you take control your body's chemistry and give yourself more energy. Even very short breath holds create slight changes in your biochemistry, increasing the amount of carbon dioxide in your blood and thereby delivering more oxygen into your brain and throughout your body.

Experiencing Rising Carbon Dioxide Levels in Your Body

That is Respiration 101, the theory. And now we are going to experience it, so it doesn't just remain book knowledge! Like we did with nitric oxide, I want you to both know and feel with your interoceptive awareness carbon dioxide in your blood. Let's experience, once again, this feeling of rising levels of carbon dioxide in our system right now:

- Inhale, then exhale and hold your breath.

- You are going to hold your breath for longer than feels comfortable.

- Relax and notice how you feel. Keep holding your breath.

- When you feel a strong urge to breathe, don't breathe immediately. Relax for a few more seconds. You are feeling carbon dioxide levels rising in your blood.

- Notice the strong urge to breathe.

- Hold your breath for one more second.

- And then inhale normally and relax.

- After a minute or two, try it again to identify that urge to breathe and feel the signals the chemoreceptors are sending to your brain telling you to breathe. That's the feeling of carbon dioxide . . . and then breathe.

The duration you hold your breath right now isn't important. What you are identifying is the distinct, urgent need to breathe. You are feeling with interoceptive awareness your body's changing chemistry. That intense feeling is undeniable and is useful in your breathing interventions, exercises, and practices. Breath holding in this book is not used as a test of your willpower. This won't become a competition. Rather, the breath holding we use in this book is used to adjust your biochemistry for your mental and physical health.

Breath holding should be approached with caution. I have had the good fortune of working with teachers and medical doctors during my hypoxic (low levels of oxygen concentration in the blood) and hypercapnic (higher levels of carbon dioxide concentration in the blood) training. Very extended breath holding should only be practiced under supervision. None of the breath holding exercises recommended in this book will send you into a hypoxic nor hypercapnic state.

Benefits of Conscious Breath Holding

Why do I call breath holding a superpower? It's because of three specific extraordinary benefits, and they all relate to entering that space between stimulus and reaction. This is about reclaiming power in our lives.

First, conscious breath holding is a pattern interrupt to incessant thought loops. I have found no other method, physical or mental, that can so quickly halt my mind. The ability to pause thinking, indeed, to stop the arising of thoughts all together, is extremely useful not only in meditation practice but also in daily life when you can't seem to stop worrying or when anxiety overcomes you. As it says in the famous treatise on yoga, *Hatha Yoga Pradipika*, "When the breath is unsteady, the mind is unsteady. When the breath is steady, the mind is steady, and the yogi becomes steady. Therefore, one should restrain the breath."[3]

The next time during your meditation practice, or during a bout of worry, try a few rounds of holding your breath for a 5 count upon exhalation (make sure it's after an exhale). This is called the Conscious Pause. Just breathe normally and after you exhale, hold your breath, and rest your attention in your body until you feel the urge to breathe, then breathe in lightly through the nose. Observe what happens. It's simple, and profound. Watch the thought-reaction-thought-reaction wheel slow and maybe come to a halt—this is the pattern interruption.

Whenever I hear a teacher say, "Wisdom lies within you," I always think of how powerful a pattern interruption is to opening that inner space for wisdom to manifest. Once after I led a teenager in this technique of short breath holds before a meditation session, he told me that "I realized that I don't have to have a strong opinion about every thought that pops in my mind." I wished I'd had that realization as a teenager.

The second benefit to breath holding is that it adds nuance and depth to the breathing dials of your nervous system. Generally, holding your breath after you inhale brings the mind into a focused and ready disposition, perhaps even an energized state. On the other end, holding your breath for a few seconds after the exhale usually slows down your mind, spreading a feeling of calm throughout your body. Experimenting with the feeling that comes from repeated holds on the inhale and/or exhale offers you a tool for concentration or relaxation.

It is worth mentioning that you can hold your breath maximally and submaximally. Maximum breath holds that challenge mental and physical fortitude with a conscious stressor may improve carbon dioxide tolerance and signal a series of physiological adaptations. We are not practicing maximal breath holds in this book—they should be learned under direct supervision of a teacher and not from a book. Breath holding after exhalation, for some individuals who are prone to anxiety attacks, might stress the system too much.

Instead, we are using submaximal breath holds that enhance mindfulness, calm an agitated mind, stimulate the parasympathetic nervous system, and have therapeutic effects such as improving immune function and increasing anti-inflammatory effects. As with most breathing practices, it is the consistency rather than intensity that delivers positive results over time. And specific to breath holding, you need to find what your minimum effective dose is to achieve your desired results.

The third benefit of breath holding comes from training in high-altitude simulation protocols, like the ones that the Oxygen Advantage teaches. These more advanced breath-holding drills used while exercising result in an increased concentration of carbon dioxide in the blood (hypercapnic), while at the same time lowering the concentration of oxygen in your blood (hypoxic). I have used this combined hypercapnic and hypoxic training specifically for mountain bike racing and tracked my improved performance, muscle recovery, and endurance.

You can begin today gaining benefits from breath holding with a practice just referred to above: the Conscious Pause. This practice involves holding the breath after a relaxed exhalation, focusing on maintaining comfort and observing the body's response. This isn't a long breath hold. You hold your breath only until you feel a light-to-moderate urge to breathe and then you inhale smooth and long through your nose. If you must gasp or take a big breath in, you've held too long.

The Conscious Pause can be done seated or walking. You'll likely hold your breath between 5 and 30 seconds. You don't need to time the duration of the pause. Rather, use your interoception to feel the signal to breathe and inhale through the nose comfortably. Repeat for five rounds. The Conscious Pause is particularly effective when done immediately before a stressful situation occurs or when you recognize you've already been provoked—it's a perfect real-time de-stressor.

I recommend using the Conscious Pause in times when you are experiencing an acute stressor and can take a moment before reacting; though sometimes we don't have the convenience of time, as action is required! You might also use the Conscious Pause immediately before a stressful situation unfolds, such as before public speaking or when low-level anxiety is brewing.

PRACTICE

The Conscious Pause

You can do the Conscious Pause while seated, lying down, or walking. Ease into any breath-holding practice—there is no need to overdo it. I do not recommend any breath-holding practices while driving or on a bicycle, or near water.

- Place your tongue on the roof of your mouth. Lips should be comfortably closed with the teeth slightly apart.

- Take a gentle and relaxed inhalation through your nose, allowing your abdomen to naturally expand.

- As you exhale through your nose, let go of any tension and release the breath completely.

- At the bottom of the exhale, hold your breath. If you wish to pinch your nose lightly, that is fine. Maintain a calm and relaxed state during this pause, focusing on the sensation of stillness.

- Allow the first signal to breathe to arise but don't breathe. Relax.

- When you feel a moderate urge to breathe, slowly and lightly breathe in through your nose with your mouth closed.

- Notice the sensation in your body and what is moving in your mind.

- If you have to gasp, take a fast quick breath, or breathe so strong that you collapsed your nostrils, you held the controlled pause too long. Go easy.

- Repeat this practice for 5 to 10 rounds.

- You may notice that your time of retention increases—but be guided by your urge to breathe.

Breath Holding as a Practice

My own breath holding practice started with my study and practice of Buddhism, yoga, and pranayama in Nepal 30 years ago. I was residing in Kathmandu at the time and working as a human rights monitor. I lived near the Pashupatinath Temple, where Hindu mendicants and yogis were residing in the nearby forest. There I met a teacher, Yogi Bharat, who introduced me to breath holding as a way to steady my mind and use it as a tool to enter nondual states of consciousness.

Yogi Bharat had been a successful businessman in Delhi earlier in his life but had renounced his material possessions after his wife died. He wandered the subcontinent to various holy sites to meditate. He spoke English perfectly. We'd meet under the banyan trees in the grounds overlooking the temple. Nearly every time he taught, he reminded me, quoting from the *Yoga Sutras*, "Yoga is the stilling of the fluctuations of the mind." This was his intention and practice, to use the body and breath to still the mind and enter profound states of meditation.

One of the first techniques Yogi Bharat taught me was breathing with equal cadence, what he called *samavritti*. *Sama* means "equal" and *vritti* means "movement," and combined the practice means to inhale, pause, exhale, and pause for the same duration of time. Samavritti practice—equal ratioed breathing—has been popularized in the West with the name *Box Breathing* or *square breathing*.

Pranayama practices are often presented with ratios, such as 1:1:1:1, where, for example, you breathe in for a 5 count, hold for 5, exhale for 5, and hold for 5. There are innumerable ratios to use depending on the desired effect and the capacity of the breather. Similar to adjusting the breathing dials on our nervous system, using specific ratios to change the pattern of inhalation and exhalation and holding the breath allows us to regulate our nervous system, or in the case of my teacher, to calm the vicissitudes of thoughts and thinking. At this point, you know that a longer exhalation than inhalation increases the parasympathetic tone, and alternatively, if you inhale for a longer count than you exhale, you stimulate your sympathetic response that tends to create focus, strong attention, and an increase in energy.

When you hold your breath after the inhalation, this tends to wake you up with energy. If you hold your breath after the exhalation, this tends to downregulate your system.[††] If you combine holds with specific ratios, you can dial up or down your nervous system. Some ratios that you can experiment might be:

Energy-boosting ratio: 2:4:1:1
Preparing-for-bed ratio: 1:1:2:2
Reducing anxiety ratio: 1:2:3:1
Box Breathing ratio: 1:1:1:1

With the energy-boosting ratio, for example, if you inhale for a 4 count, you will hold for 8 count, exhale for a 2 count, and hold for 2. Or, for the preparing-for-bed ratio, you inhale for 3, hold for 3, exhale for a 6 count, and hold for a 6 count. Remembering that emphasizing inhalation and holding at the top increases sympathetic drive, while elongating exhales and holds afterward moves you toward parasympathetic response. Empower yourself by experimenting with ratio breathing and breath holds to find what works for your nervous system.

Let's return to equal ratio (1:1:1:1) breathing or Box Breathing. Because you are holding your breath in equal ratios, the effect is usually both refreshing and calming.

[††] Holding the breath in pranayama is always accompanied with the application of internal locks, or *bandhas*. The three principal locks are engaging the *mulabhanda* at the perineum to contain and push the energy upward; pulling the navel up and toward the spine, known as *uddihana bhanda*, to push the energy upward; and lowering the chin onto the notch in your sternum, known as the *jhalandara bandha*, to push the energy down. Working with these internal locks and breath holding on the inhale or exhale, the practice contains your vital energy—prana—in the central channel.

You'll need to find your own count that will work for your ratio, one that does not create a feeling of breathlessness when you do the practice for 5 to 10 minutes. For most people, this will be either a 3 or 4 count. We'll use a 4 count for the practice below.

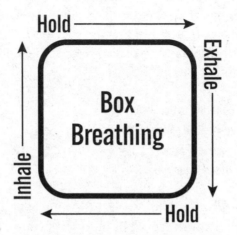

PRACTICE

Box Breathing

- Assume a comfortable position: seated, lying down, or walking.

- Place one hand on your sternum and the other on your belly.

- Set your intention, thinking: *May this Box Breathing practice empower me with clarity and patience.*

- Turn your attention to your breath for a moment and practice breath awareness. No need to change, just notice how you are breathing this moment.

- Breathe slowly in and out of your nose.

- During Box Breathing, there should not be any strain. Just relax, mentally counting.

- Let's begin to box breathe.

- Breathe in comfortably through the nose for a count of 4.

- Hold your breath at the top for a count of 4. Relax your shoulders.

- Release the breath hold and exhale out the nose for a count of 4.

- After you exhale, hold your breath for a count of 4. Relax your face.

- Inhale for a 4 count and continue Box Breathing for 5 to 10 minutes.

- At the conclusion, let go of the Box Breathing and notice for a minute or so how your body and mind feel.

If you find yourself breathless while doing this practice, feel tension arising in the body, or have the need to take extra breaths, you are overextending. You might decrease strength of the breath or reduce it to a 3:3:3:3 count. Feel free to experiment with different ratios as this will give you experiential know-how in adjusting your breathing cadence and length of breath holds for desired effects.

For more visually inclined individuals, visualize a box during the practice. On the inhale, follow the vertical axis upward. During the retention, count while moving horizontally. On the exhale, move down the side of the box. And on the hold, complete the box. Keep the count equal.

KEY INSIGHTS

- Conscious breath holding is a superpower because it is a pattern interrupt to thought loops, providing you the space to respond appropriately rather than react habitually to stressful situations. Breath holding is your fourth tool in your breathing tool kit.

- The Conscious Pause is a particularly effective breathing intervention in preparation for stressful situations or after you have been provoked.

- Holding your breath after an inhalation dials up your energy. Holding your breath after an exhalation downregulates your system.

Chapter 6

INTEGRATING AIR

Using your breath to adjust your nervous system, to breathe how you want to feel, requires your attention, openness, and a willingness to adapt to the ups and downs in your life. In a word, this is called *integrating*.

Integration is weaving your experiential knowledge, intuitive understanding, and the actual breathing interventions into the fabric of your daily life. Integration is how you embody knowledge, incubating it within yourself so that it becomes a lived wisdom.

I'm not suggesting your breath practice become another lifestyle hack to fit between your job, workout, taking care of your family, and all the rest—though if you are into lifestyle hacks, go for it. You don't need to fly off for weekend breath retreats in Tulum or Ojai—though if you have the means, go for it. And you certainly don't need a guru to give you permission to do any breathing practice—though if you have a guru, make sure you have chosen wisely.

Instead, what I'm encouraging you to do is partner with your breath throughout the day and night. Marry your spacious awareness with the ebb and flow of your breath, letting the breath breathe you. This is the essence of breath awareness. With interoception—not just the

intellect—sense your interiority and start a breathing intervention if needed. This is taking back the command over
your nervous system that chronic stress has usurped from
you. Be patient in learning how adjusting the strength,
pace, and volume of your breathing turns the dials and
regulates your nervous system. You have the power. And
remember, if you are a mouth breather, switch to nasal
breathing; it is the single most significant thing you can
do right now to upgrade your well-being. Make sure you
are breathing through your nose while sleeping—it is of
paramount significance. Stay curious and playful in discovering breathing interventions that work for you. Your
breath is always there for you, the most loyal of compan-
ions in life.

Mnemonic Nose Breathing

To integrate AIR into your daily life, especially when
you feel stress or anxiety, I suggest you create your own
breathing integration practice called Mnemonic Nose
Breathing. *Mnemonic* is a word that refers to a memory aid
or technique. In this practice, there are three steps.

Step 1 is to place the tongue in a relaxed manner on
the upper palate, with the tip of the tongue just behind
(but not touching) the teeth. Keep your lips closed without strain in the jaw.

Step 2 is to inhale and exhale lightly through your nose.

Step 3 is to silently repeat your chosen positive affirmation or mantra.

These three steps, placement of the tongue, nose breathing, and mantra constitute Mnemonic Nose Breathing.

The reason to have this practice is because stressful
situations are guaranteed in life, so you might as well have

a planned response. The Stoics called this *premeditatio malorum*, premeditation on troubles, which encourages us to anticipate and mentally prepare for the challenges that lie ahead. When we embrace premeditatio malorum, we acknowledge that difficulties are an inevitable part of life's journey, and, importantly, we have a planned response. This is taking part in our own rescue rather than waiting for outside conditions to change. By having a plan of action and then responding appropriately, we are reframing our stress response so that stress is a reminder of our capacity.[‡‡] In other words, let stress be a reminder that you are resilient and that you've got this!

You might ask, why bring the tongue into this? The position of your tongue plays a significant role in nasal breathing because it fully opens your airway.

Try this right now: spread your tongue on the roof of your mouth and breathe through your nose. Easy, right?

Now, try this: keep your tongue on the roof of your mouth, pinch your nose, and breathe through your mouth. Nope, it can't be done.

When you spread your tongue on the roof of your mouth, the only option is to breathe through your nose. As soon as you place your tongue in the anatomically optimal breathing position, nasal breathing starts, your vagus nerve is stimulated, and these signals remind your brain that all is safe, and you can relax.

If you are a habitual mouth breather and your tongue regularly sags to the bottom of your mouth, you don't have to worry because the tongue is trainable. It just takes a little mindfulness and effort.

[‡‡]   For other reframing techniques, see Elissa Epel, Ph.D., *The Stress Prescription: 7 Days to More Joy and Ease* (New York: Penguin Books, 2022). Also, see Jamieson et al., "Turning the Knots in Your Stomach into Bows; Reappraising Arousal Improves Performance on GRE," *Journal of Experimental Social Psychology* 46, no. 1 (Jan 2010).

When you place the tongue on the roof of your mouth, this is the reminder to breathe slowly in and out of the nose. Step 1 and 2—tongue position and nasal breathing—of Mnemonic Nose Breathing, happen in quick succession and create a physiologically agile and open state.

Step 3 is to repeat or recall a phrase or word that is associated with the way you want to feel. For some these words may be a mantra or prayer, while for others it may be an affirmation or positive self-talk. What we tell ourselves, how we frame our situation in life, the lens through which we choose to look either exacerbates or deescalates our stress. When you repeat a mantra or positive affirmation, you are creating a pattern of thought and behavior in the mind. This is massively significant because repeated thoughts arising in your mind, the Ferris wheel of patterned thinking, is the most common of internal stressors, according to stress researchers. Mantras and positive affirmations not only function as a pattern interruption to negative thought loops but allow for a new lens through which you see yourself and the world around you. When you change the way you see the world, when you change what you are telling yourself, the world itself changes.

Right now, choose a word or short phrase that feels empowering and resonates with what you want to create within yourself and manifest in the world. This is your mantra or positive affirmation for today and tomorrow. Your mantra or positive affirmation may be a reframing of negative self-talk. It may be celebrating who you already are. It may be what you are becoming. Keep it concise and personal. I recommend words that are affirming rather than aspirational; for example, rather than "I want to be joyful," choose "I am joyful" or another "I am . . ." statement. Go ahead and jot your mantra down on paper.

PRACTICE

Mnemonic Nose Breathing

- Assume a comfortable position: seated, lying down, or walking.

- Place one hand on your belly if that feels reassuring.

- My mantra or positive affirmation for today is: _____.

- Step 1. Tongue. Place the tongue in a relaxed manner on the roof of your mouth, behind but not touching your teeth.

- Step 2. Nasal Breathing. Breathe slowly in and out of the nose.

- There need not be any strain. Just relax.

- Step 3. Mantra. Repeat your mantra or positive affirmation once on the inhale and once on the exhale.

- Breathe in, silently repeating your word or phrase.

- Relax and breathe out, silently repeating your word or phrase.

- Continue for a few minutes.

- At the conclusion, let go of the practice and notice for a minute or so how your body and mind feel.

Combining nasal breathing with positive affirmations is a powerful way to regulate your nervous system as it works simultaneously on your physiological, psychological, and spiritual being. Regularly practiced, the release of stress hormones in your body are reduced. You feel more at ease, accepting of what is out of your control, and empowered to act upon what is in your control. And you are cultivating your inner landscape.

Integrating Conscious Breathing Throughout the Day

In addition to Mnemonic Nose Breathing as a regular integrative practice, here are a few other reminders for how to integrate the breath into your daily life.

1. *Breathing Yourself Awake with Light*—upon waking, go outside (or open a window to your home) and breathe with direct sunlight on your face and skin. If possible, breathe with your bare feet on the earth. Let your intuition guide how you breathe at the start of the day. Your diaphragm will love a little massage too!

2. *Breathing with Gratitude*—while you are preparing your coffee or tea, let the hot drink be a reminder to breathe deeply with gratitude. Think of at least one thing you are grateful for and how you'll reciprocate that feeling of joy. Holding that thought, do a few rounds of Box Breathing.

3. *Breath Refreshers*—when you feel low, frustrated, have brain fog, or are in any other state you want to change, take a break to breathe. Remember the acronym AIR: check in with breath awareness, initiate a breathing intervention to adjust the dials on your nervous system, and regulate as needed throughout the day.

4. *Breath Emergency Plan*—have a plan for when anxiety spikes or an acute stressful situation hits. What breathing interventions work for you? It need not be complicated, but have it at the ready so that your breathing tool kit becomes second nature. I suggest either 4:6 Cadence Breathing, the Conscious Pause, or Mnemonic Nose Breathing. Physiological Sighs work almost immediately.

5. *Breathe Through Your Nose*—keep it nasal. Now that you have read this far, you will reflexively notice when you are mouth breathing. Take a mental note of the situations you are in when you are mouth breathing—those may be threatening or fear-inducing scenarios. Return to breathing through your nose throughout the day. And smile each time you remember.

6. *Breathing for Digestion*—so that you extract nutrition from your food and digest it properly, prepare your belly before eating. Spend a few minutes on extended exhalations or any other parasympathetic-inducing intervention until you feel salvia forming in your mouth, at which time you'll know it's time to eat. Massage your palate and inner lips with your tongue. You can do this while you are preparing food to save time, but be sure to sit down to eat. Chew slowly.

7. *Breath and Movement*—exercise, every day. Find whatever movements you enjoy and pay attention to your breath when you exercise. If it is not high-intensity exercise, keep it nasal.

If you exercise in a gym, great; if at home, awesome; if it's in nature, even better!

8. *Breathing in the Evening*—get outside and breathe as the sun is going down at dusk—even for just a few minutes. This will help establish your circadian rhythm with the release of melatonin in your system. Practice long exhales with the setting sun.

9. *Breathing and Sleep*—keep your mouth closed while sleeping, using mouth tape or a chin strap, to fully restore your body during the night. While lying in bed, lightly place your attention and extend your exhalation. Humming before bed is a somatic lullaby.

10. *Breathing with Challenges*—consciously challenge yourself physically every day. You need not exhaust or overwhelm yourself, but rather, move outside of your comfort zone and ride the wave of the challenge with your breath. Feel your edges every day. You got this!

KEY INSIGHTS

- By integrating your experiential insights, intuition, and breathing techniques, you gain control over your emotional, physical, and spiritual well-being. Integration of AIR—awareness, intervention, and regulation—is the fifth tool in your breathing tool kit.

- Mnemonic Nose Breathing is a planned practice to meet life's inevitable challenges and stress. To self-regulate and improve resilience, place your tongue on the upper palate, breathe lightly through the nose, and silently repeat a positive affirmation or mantra—this is Mnemonic Nose Breathing.

- Breathing how you want to feel is taking personal responsibility for your state of mind.

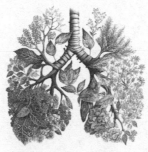

BREATHE HOW YOU WANT TO LIVE

Chapter 7

IDENTIFYING
DYSFUNCTIONAL
BREATHING

You now have a grasp on the principles of optimal breathing. Your breathing tool kit is always at the ready so you can adjust the breathing dials on your nervous system when needed. In Part II, we are going to refine and sharpen these breathing tools so that you become even more resilient and agile in daily life—for exercise, meditation, sleep, and when put in acute stressful situations. In essence, we are applying the breathing tool kit from Part I to life.

To do so, we need to assess if you have any dysfunctional breathing mechanics—that is, if the way you breathe day-to-day is less than optimal. After assessing if you have any dysfunctional breathing mechanics, you'll learn ways to correct yourself by optimizing the use of your nose, tongue, diaphragm, and other parts of your respiratory system. This allows you to be in command of your respiratory biochemistry, the inner secret to breathing how you want to feel.

Dysfunctional breathing is breathing in a way that is inefficient or inappropriate for the current state of your metabolic demands. Another way to state this is that breathing is suboptimal when the way you breathe prevents your system from having the oxygen supply your brain and muscles need. Dysfunctional breathing holds you back from manifesting the best version of yourself.

It is estimated that as high as 50 to 80 percent of adults have some degree of dysfunctional breathing.[1] Causes of this dysfunction include chronic overbreathing, mouth breathing, poor head and shoulder posture from computers and smartphone use, chronic stress, and sedentary lifestyles. Physical challenges such as a deviated septum might also create dysfunctional breathing, as can hormonal changes and the aging process.

It's likely you have some degree of dysfunctional breathing if you exhibit any of these symptoms or behaviors:

1. Breathing through your mouth regularly

2. Poor sleep quality, sleep apnea, or snoring

3. Waking up with dry mouth or lips

4. Feeling tired and fatigued in the morning

5. Unconsciously holding your breath

6. Chronic nasal congestion

7. Shortness of breath when walking or climbing stairs

8. Poor digestion

9. Frequent yawning and sighing throughout the day

10. Audible breathing sounds

11. Regular lower-back pain

12. Frequent urination during the night

13. Brain fog and difficulty concentrating

14. Low Body Oxygen Limit Test (BOLT) score—
    you'll learn to assess your BOLT shortly

Why Breathing Too Much Air Is Unhealthy

The main characteristic of dysfunctional breathing is breathing too much air. You may wonder, "What is the problem with breathing too much? Won't I just get more oxygen?"

Another name for breathing too much is hyperventilation, which we touched on earlier. Hyperventilation happens when you breathe out more carbon dioxide than is necessary to keep your body healthy. This kind of breathing may cause dizziness, lightheadedness, numbness or tingling sensations, palpitations, chest tightness, and even panic attacks. You're not getting more oxygen when you are breathing shallow and fast; rather, you are blowing off too much carbon dioxide. Remember, cardon dioxide is the stimulus for oxygen to be released into your tissues. It might seem counterintuitive, but your brain and body don't receive the needed delivery of oxygen when you breathe too much air.

When someone is panicking and huffing and puffing in distress, they are hyperventilating. And what did your grandmother do when this happened? She gave the person a paper bag and told them to breathe into it. Why did this calm the person down? Because from within the paper bag, the hyperventilating person breathed back in higher concentrations of carbon dioxide that they had just expelled, which caused oxygen to be released into their brain and body.

While you might not think you regularly hyperventilate, there is a spectrum to hyperventilation. You may not need to breathe regularly into a paper bag, which is at the high end of the hyperventilating spectrum, but if you have any of the previous symptoms, you are likely on the lower end of hyperventilation—and this we are calling *overbreathing*.

Overbreathing is when you breathe too much air, too quickly, too often. As Patrick McKeown of Oxygen Advantage says, "Just as we have an optimal quantity of water and food to consume each day, we also have an optimal quantity of air to breathe. And just as eating too much damages our health, so can overbreathing."[2]

We average 10 to 14 breaths per minute. Pause right now and count the number of breaths in the next minute—go ahead, try it. Look at a second hand on a clock or open your timer and count when you inhale and exhale—that's one. Count how many times you breathe per minute without consciously changing your cadence or pattern.

If you breathe more than 14 breaths per minute, you are overbreathing.

Overbreathers tend to breathe about 15 breaths or more every minute when they are relaxing, often with the mouth open, which means they breathe some 10,000 to 20,000 more breaths per day than normal. The consequences of breathing 30,000 to 40,000 times a day negatively impacts the efficiency of your respiratory, cardiovascular, and nervous systems. This is because overbreathing leads to a disruption in the balance of carbon dioxide and oxygen in the blood. This imbalance, as alluded to earlier, reduces blood flow to vital organs and tissue and oxygen delivery to the cells. Additionally, it tells your body that there is danger near, and adrenaline and noradrenaline are released into your system. Overbreathing is like having an

IV drip of stress hormones pumped throughout your body all day long.

Why Do We Breathe through Our Mouths?

The primary reason we overbreathe boils down to one dysfunctional pattern: mouth breathing. I know we discussed mouth breathing earlier, but its negative impact on our health cannot be overstated. The reasons you might be a mouth breather are likely complex and a combination of medical reasons such as asthma or sinusitis; a structural challenge such as a deviated septum; and/or psychological reasons such as chronic stress or PTSD that keep your sympathetic nervous system switched on all the time.[§§]

If you are chronically stressed, or experiencing depression or bouts of anxiety, you are more likely to resort to mouth breathing. There is a symbiotic relationship between mouth breathing, poor mechanics, and challenging emotional states, and it isn't always clear which is causing the other. What is clear in the research, however, is that by correcting the mechanics of breathing—starting by switching from using the mouth to the nose for breathing—you position yourself in a more psychologically advantageous position to deal with stress.

Mouth breathing is a habit. Once the mouth breathing habit is formed, it takes discipline to retrain yourself to be a nasal breather, but it is a habit worth changing. Failing to breathe through the nose eventuates in a decline in the extraordinary functioning of the nasal passage itself and the muscles associated with breathing. Use it or lose it!

Mouth breathers tend to take shallow breaths using secondary respiratory muscles in the upper chest. Overuse

---

[§§] If you have a structural issue that prevents any nasal breathing at all, it's essential to seek professional help to restore it and mitigate the harmful effects of mouth breathing.

or extended reliance on these secondary muscles leads to their tightening. This contrasts with nasal breathers who use the primary respiratory muscle, the diaphragm, which pulls the air lower in the lungs. The cascade of negative effects when your day-to-day breathing—seated, walking casually, light exercise—is done through the mouth, include:

- Expelling too much carbon dioxide, which decreases oxygen delivery to your brain and muscles

- Increasing the tidal volume of air that causes imbalance of oxygen and carbon dioxide

- Stimulating your sympathetic nervous system, keeping you constantly on guard

- Increasing upper-chest movement that weakens your core stability, causing back pain

- Constricting your smooth muscles surrounding blood vessels and airways

- Limiting physical capacity and enjoyment for sports and exercise

- Setting you up for poor sleep quality

- Promoting overbreathing

Consequences from overbreathing impact all your body's systems. Your cardiovascular system is taxed, leading to palpitations, missed beats, cold hands and feet, and capillary vasoconstriction. Neurologically, it can cause dizziness, brain fog, feeling faint without actually fainting, and headaches. The respiratory system goes into overdrive, resulting in shortness of breath, an irritating cough, chest tightness, air hunger, an inability to take a deep breath, and excessive sighing, yawning, and sniffing. Muscularly, overbreathing may cause cramps and muscle pain in the neck, shoulders, and lower back (due to lack of core stability). Psychologically, overbreathing leads to tension, anxiety, and panic. It might also exacerbate allergies and cause gastrointestinal difficulties, gastric reflux, dry mouth and throat, acid regurgitation, heartburn, flatulence, belching, air swallowing, and abdominal discomfort. Overall, overbreathing contributes to weakness, exhaustion, suboptimal concentration, impaired memory and performance, and disturbed sleep.[3]

Assessing Your Breathing with the Body Oxygen Level Test (BOLT)

Another way to assess if you are overbreathing or if there are other suboptimal breathing mechanics is to take the Body Oxygen Level Test (BOLT) score. Researchers for more than 50 years have known that the length of time you can comfortably hold your breath is a marker for functional breathing. I learned of the BOLT test in my training with the Oxygen Advantage when I became an advanced instructor. I regularly teach this to track progress in upgrading breathing mechanics and efficiency, and I perform it almost daily myself.

While there is some subjectivity to this test, other ways to measure your sensitivity to carbon dioxide involve spending time in a laboratory or wearing a capnometer, both of which I have found fascinating to do but are impractical daily. Here, instead, you use your BOLT score for feedback as you improve upon and retrain your breathing mechanics. I recommend taking the BOLT first thing in the morning before exercise or caffeine, at the same time each day, so that you track your progress as you work toward breathing optimally.

Your BOLT score is assessed by holding your breath after you exhale and timing how many seconds until you feel the first urge to breathe. Importantly, this is not a test to see how long you can hold your breath. Let me repeat that: this is not a breath-holding contest. There is no will-power involved with the BOLT. Rather, you are measuring the time it takes for your body to urge you, "Hey, take a breath." Listen to your body.

When you hold your breath after your exhale for the BOLT score, what do you "feel" when your body signals you to breathe? Probably one of these:

- The need to swallow

- Constriction in the throat

- Your throat or diaphragm involuntarily contracts

When you feel one of these signals to breathe, note the number of seconds that elapsed and breathe normally. When you resume breathing, it should be absolutely normal. If you must breathe deeply or have any breathlessness or gasping, you went past the first urge to breathe. It is best to perform the BOLT score after you have been seated and resting for 5 to 10 minutes and with your heart rate normal.

Let's find your BOLT score now. Read the instructions first, and then perform it. Have a watch with a second hand or stopwatch ready to use.

PRACTICE

Body Oxygen Level Test

To ascertain an accurate score, rest seated for 5 to 10 minutes before taking the BOLT.

- Take a few normal breaths in and out through your nose.

- Relax as you are breathing.

- Breathe in normally through the nose.

- Breathe out normally through the nose.

- After a normal nasal exhalation, hold your nose closed with your fingers to stop breathing.

- Start your timer.

- Time the number of seconds until you feel the first definite urge to breathe.

- When you feel the first urge to breathe, stop the timer.

- Let go and breathe normally through the nose.

- Resume normal breathing.

- Your inhalation after the breath hold should be calm. If you had to take a deep breath, gasp, or were otherwise strained on the inhale, you went past the first urge to breathe. Wait a minute and retake the BOLT.

What does your BOLT score indicate?

Below 10 seconds: Your day-to-day breathing is likely audible to others, irregular, and strained, with repeated sighing and yawning during the day; your sleep is disturbed by apnea and a frequent need to urinate, especially at night;

and you feel tired in the morning. You may unconsciously hold your breath during the day. Your physical and emotional health is probably impacted by dysfunctional breathing, including constant breathlessness or feelings of panic or anxiety. Increasing your BOLT score will have noticeable physical and cognitive benefits.

10 to 20 seconds: You likely have chronically blocked sinuses with frequent wheezing or coughing. Your sleep is disrupted, and your focus, concentration, and energy are not sustainable. You likely become short of breath quickly with light exercise, are unable take a deep and satisfying breath, and may feel anxious easily. For every 5 seconds your BOLT score increases, you will feel a significant boost in your overall energy, less breathlessness during the day and while exercising, and an elevated mood.

20 to 30 seconds: Your day-to-day breathing is likely calm and not audible and does not take effort. When your exercise level increases, you likely resort to mouth breathing immediately. Your BOLT score is good, but there are many health and fitness benefits still available if you improve your score. Keep it nasal all the time except during intense exercise.

30 to 40 seconds: Your sensitivity to carbon dioxide is low and indicates a strong cardiovascular system, your sleep is likely restorative, and your exercise endurance is excellent. It's time to incorporate high-altitude simulation into your fitness regime.

Our body's sensitivity to carbon dioxide is one significant determinate of our health, affecting nearly every aspect of how our body functions. Improved breathing with a lower sensitivity to carbon dioxide ensures that all the interrelated psychophysical parts of ourselves function in harmony, allowing us to achieve our maximum potential in body and mind.

A significant number of people I work with begin with a low BOLT score, around 10 seconds, especially if they have asthma, sinusitis, or regularly experience anxiety or panic. Even athletes who are in fine physical shape may have a BOLT score between 10 to 20 seconds because of dysfunctional breathing patterns. The upside of having a low BOLT score is you have a clear pathway for the need to use your breathing tool kit from this book.

The obvious question arises, "How do I increase my BOLT score?" The answer is to fold your breathing tool kit from Part I into your life. This includes correcting any dysfunctional breathing that you may have and that begins with habitually nasal breathing; correct tongue posture; using your diaphragm, intercostals, and levatores as the primary breathing muscle; and regular conscious breath holding practice, like the Conscious Pause or Box Breathing.

What Kind of Breather Are You?

We all have our unique ways of breathing, and it can change depending on physical and mental stress, intensity of exercise, posture, and age. It's beneficial if we become familiar with what type of default breather we are in our day-to-day life because it gives us insight into any needed adjustments. Correcting dysfunction in our normal breathing is the starting point because we carry our unconscious habits into how we breathe when acute stressors hit, during exercise, public speaking, meditation, and other life situations.

The optimal mechanics of breathing look like a gentle wave starting in the lower abdomen and moving outward and upward. It's the way an infant breathes when they are sleeping, or like a healthy dog, where the inhalation gracefully fills the abdomen and then opens the rib basket. And the exhale glides out, no force is required. There are smooth pauses as the breath transitions between inhalation and exhalation, a natural rhythm at play.

Let's take a closer look at your own breathing style. After you read the descriptions below, have a look in a mirror for a few minutes at the movements of your torso when you are breathing. Or video yourself. Just breathe normally and observe if you are nose or mouth breathing, and if and when your belly, ribs, and shoulders move. It's possible that you fall into a combination of one or more of these descriptions:

> ***Chest Breather***—the distinguishing characteristics are the inhalation initiates in the upper chest, resulting in the shoulders moving up and down, which is why this is sometimes known as "vertical breathing." Often there is an exaggerated outward-puffing superhero-like chest, while the abdomen remains relatively immobile. To compensate for this style, chest breathers rely heavily on secondary breathing muscles located in the upper chest, back, and shoulders. This reliance leads to stiffness, tension, and discomfort in these areas, as well as in the lower back, which is often overly arched. Chest breathers tend to maintain constant stiffness and bracing in their stomach muscles, sometimes from the habit of keeping the belly sucked in. This is one of the most prevalent forms of dysfunctional breathing.
>
> ***Unconscious Breath Holder***—the defining characteristic is unconsciously holding the breath. This breathing interruption can occur during inhalation, exhalation, or in between breaths, and it is

often accompanied by physical and mental tension. The chest breather and the breath holder are the most prevalent forms of dysfunctional breathing. In the next chapter, you'll delve deeper into the topic of unconscious breath holding. Unconscious breath holders often only realize they have stopped breathing when a big sigh or gasp overcomes them, often with an increased heart rate following. Blood oxygen levels may drop to unhealthy levels before the gasp reflex kicks in, as if a stranglehold has been released. There are often underlying psychological factors contributing to this breathing dysfunction that may include long-term or chronic stress responses, past trauma, or a sense of perceived threat.

Paradoxical Breather—the distinguishing characteristic is during inhalation, the abdomen pulls inward toward the spine, which is the opposite of the optimal pattern. Ideally, on the inhale, the diaphragm descends, and the abdomen expands outward. However, when a paradoxical breather pulls the belly in on the inhale, it creates an active resistance against the diaphragm and doesn't allow for a satisfying inhalation. This leads to chronic tension caused by breathing. Paradoxical breathers often exhibit other traits, such as initiating inhalation in the upper chest, lifting the shoulders, puffing the chest, and potential muscle tension in the neck. This habitual form of breathing usually requires dedicated practice sessions over a period of weeks or months to untrain.

Almost Breather—the distinguishing characteristic is the breath pauses after a slight inhale or exhale, lingering in a state of respiratory limbo.

Unlike the natural pause that occurs at the top of the inhale and the bottom of the exhale, the almost breather unconsciously interrupts the rhythm, sometimes multiple times, on the inhale and exhale. The halting breath causes the almost breather to sip air. The almost breather often develops this pattern due to deep traumatic events in their past, with chronic fear being a common underlying factor.

Belly-Only Breather—the distinctive characteristic is that the movement of the breath originates and remains confined to the lower abdomen. The movement of the ribs is either minimal or nonexistent. As a result, the belly forcefully protrudes forward, often causing an exaggerated curvature in the lower back that can develop into weakness. Belly-only breathers tend to rely on secondary breathing muscles, such as the transverse abdominis, rectus abdominis, and internal and external obliques, to forcefully push the belly outward during inhalation. These muscles should not be responsible for initiating the breath but rather remain relaxed and elastic. Belly-only breathers often experience a loss of mobility in their rib cage and may develop lower-back pain.

Breath Controller—the defining characteristic is either pushing the exhale out or stopping the exhalation before it has completed itself. In our natural breathing, the exhale effortlessly falls out as the diaphragm elastically returns to its resting position, requiring minimal energy. However, the breath controller unconsciously interferes with this smooth exhale by introducing a gripping sensation in the throat. While consciously controlled exhalations are effectively utilized in specific pranayama practices, such as very long exhales, or techniques employed in weightlifting to enhance intra-abdominal pressure, involuntarily applying brakes to normal exhales causes unnecessary stress, impeding the release and relaxation. The tendency to control the exhalation may originate from psychological factors, such as a perceived loss of control in one's life. Additionally, it can become a habitual pattern developed from yogic breathing, particularly the Ujjayi breathing technique.

Breath Wave Breather—this is our desired default breathing pattern. Below, we will explore two forms of the breath wave for practice that I encourage everyone to do to create muscle and neurological patterning of this rhythmic expansion and contraction. Essentially, the breath wave involves diaphragmatic breathing, where the visible movement begins in the navel area and expands outward and upward to widen the rib basket. In deeper breaths, after the wave fills the lower torso, it extends slightly into the chest and under the clavicles. In everyday situations, the breath wave primarily moves the belly and lower ribs, with no movement of the shoulders.

Correcting Dysfunctional Breathing

So let's get right into the nuts and bolts—or as the case may be, the nose and diaphragm—of functional breathing mechanics.

The first step for correcting the mechanics of over-breathing is straightforward: keep your mouth closed and breathe through your nose. You learned in Chapter 4 that nasal breathing (almost) all the time is optimal because it purifies and conditions the air you breathe before it enters your lungs, and you gain the many vasodilating and bronchodilation benefits of nitric oxide. And you know why sleeping with your mouth closed is so important, which is why you are now mouth taping.

Nasal breathing also protects your lower back and spine by pressurizing and stabilizing your entire core. Your respiratory diaphragm and back health are intricately linked. Optimal breathing mechanics aid in shaping your posture while dysfunctional breathing contributes to pain and motor control deficiency, often resulting in dysfunctional movement patterns.[4,¶¶]

Now that you've started to notice when you mouth breathe, you may find a voice in your head reminding you—*keep it nasal*. This is a wise voice!

You also may have started noticing others breathing with their mouths open while at the supermarket, walking around your neighborhood or at the airport, or especially at the gym. As you move throughout your day, let those be reminders to close your own mouth and breathe slowly. If you have the habit of mouth breathing, try taping your lips closed when watching TV or when you are on the computer. If you become winded while walking the dog or while buying groceries, slow your pace and draw long, slow breaths in and out of your nose rather than opening your mouth to breathe. When you are talking to your friends or on a video call online, try taking nasal breaths in between sentences

---

¶¶   Your respiratory diaphragm's ligaments connect to the spinal column at both the thoracic (T12) vertebrae and your lumbar (L1 and L2) vertebrae, joining it to both the middle and the lower back. Breathing problems increase the risk of back pain, and vice versa.

instead of breathing through your mouth—you'll often find those listening to you will lean toward you during the slight pause, waiting for you to speak! Begin to habituate yourself to nose breathing all the time, except when you are physically exerting yourself intensely.

Tongue

Before we move to the most important muscle for breathing, your diaphragm, another anatomical element is critical to functional breathing, and we want to explore it—your tongue. We discussed tongue position earlier during Mnemonic Nose Breathing as a breathing intervention practice. But where your tongue rests during the day and night impacts how you breathe overall, your posture, mood, and oral hygiene.[5]

When I was 12 years old, my dentist noticed my dysfunctional breathing pattern due to tongue thrusting. When I swallowed, which all of us do about 1,200 times a day, my tongue pushed forward against my bottom teeth, causing me to swallow with my mouth open. Additionally, my tongue habitually rested on the bottom of my mouth, which led to slouched shoulders and a head position that jutted forward—and I didn't even have smartphone viewing to blame! When I look at old photos from this age, I see my mouth agape in many of them. Thankfully, my dentist recognized the issue because tongue thrusting leads to buck teeth in the short term. And the tongue resting on the bottom of the mouth encourages mouth breathing, which has dire outcomes for children.

Dr. Steven Lin writes in *The Dental Diet: The Surprising Link between Your Teeth, Real Food, and Life-Changing Natural Health* about the serious health consequences for children from mouth breathing and other dysfunctional breathing patterns, which include:

1. Abnormal facial and dental development, including crowded teeth and malocclusions, leading to adaptations that reduce nasal airway function, further promoting mouth breathing

2. Narrowing and vaulting of the palate that leads to, among other things, a deviated septum

3. Increased risk of infections and illnesses, including colds and ear infections

4. Stunted speech and cognitive development

5. Tooth decay and loss

6. Poor sleep because of snoring, sleep apnea, and restlessness

7. Behavioral issues and ADHD-like symptoms

8. Difficulty concentrating

9. Poor sports performance and decreased endurance[6]

To correct my tongue thrusting, my parents and dentist enlisted a speech therapist, who put me through drills to train my tongue using muscle memory. The therapist told me it was like gym class for my tongue and had me repeatedly press the tip of my tongue behind my upper front teeth, broadening and suctioning my tongue to my palate and pulling down to make a popping sound. This is called palatal suction. My homework was to spread my tongue across the upper palate repeatedly throughout the day, with my lips closed and jaw relaxed. This helped train my tongue and jaw muscles. Not only did the drills and suctioning correct my tongue thrusting and retrain my tongue posture, it also widened my palate, which had begun to vault.

When the tongue rests on the upper palate, the airway in the back of your throat is open. If your tongue collapses down to the bottom of your mouth, the back of your tongue sags backward and obstructs the airway, causing wheezing and a chronic but subtle feeling of a chokehold. Breathing through your nose while having your tongue resting or spread across the upper palate (but not touching the teeth) should be the default position. This is the correct oral resting posture when your mouth is not eating, talking, or drinking. Strengthen your tongue with the exercise below.

PRACTICE

Tongue Strengthening

- Place the tip of your tongue behind your front teeth in the place it touches when you say, "Nah, nah, nah."

- Broaden your tongue across your upper palate, not touching your teeth, and create suction.

- Pop or click your tongue from the suction—without moving your chin. It helps to do this looking in the mirror.

- Begin with 20 reps and work your way to clicking 100 times per day.

- When your tongue fatigues, the sound will likely change and your chin will start to move, so pause and rest if you notice that happening.

Another reason the placement of your tongue is important is because the tongue and the vagus nerve have an intimate connection. A portion of the vagus nerve is located on the roof of the mouth, behind the front teeth. When you place the tongue correctly, you stimulate the vagus nerve, and this activates your body's relaxation response. This results in a calming effect that helps reduce stress levels and create a sense of safety and security.

The next time you are provoked, say when someone cuts you off in traffic, a work colleague does something annoying, your child is having a meltdown, or your cat or dog makes a mess, softly position your tongue on your upper palate and exhale long. Give it a try and add this to your breathing tool kit. Practicing mindful tongue placement is an effective way to promote relaxation, which you can do when stressed, before eating, or as you lay down to sleep.

The Buddha taught a similar technique to calm an agitated mind by pressing the tongue forcefully on the roof of the mouth.*** One of my first Buddhist meditation teachers encouraged me to rest my tongue on the upper palate, not to control my mind or stimulate the flow of energy, but rather to maintain absolute physical stillness during hours-long seated meditation. With the tongue in this position, saliva flows down the throat naturally without any need to swallow, which would otherwise cause a movement of the mouth and face. Such tongue placement is useful for achieving stillness and effective for quickly calming a restless mind.

*** The Buddha likely learned a variety of ways to use the tongue in meditation, including the advanced yogic technique of *khechari mudra*, where the tip of the tongue moves to far back of the throat and pushes on energetic points (done often while you are standing on your head) to effect deep meditative states.

It should be noted that some individuals may encounter challenges when attempting to position their tongue against the roof of their mouth. In some cases, the frenulum, which is the tissue connecting the underside of the tongue to the floor of the mouth, may be too short to allow the tongue to reach the roof of the mouth, a condition often referred to as a "tongue-tie." Additionally, some individuals may have tongue ties on the sides, inhibiting the tongue's ability to contact the roof of the mouth.

If you find it difficult to place your tongue on the palate, I recommend seeking the expertise of an orofacial myofunctional therapist or speak to your dentist. These professionals specialize in assessing tongue mobility and can offer guidance on appropriate exercises or procedures to address any limitations you may be experiencing.

Diaphragmatic Breathing with the Breath Wave

The diaphragm is your body's ultimate multitasker because it plays vital roles in breathing, posture stability, proper digestion and excretion, circulation, sexual function, and state regulation. As Dr. Belisa Vranich writes in *Breathing for Warriors,* "Reversing dysfunctional mechanics in order to give the diaphragm its throne back as a primary breathing muscle has mind-blowing health and performance consequences."[7]

We practiced diaphragmatic breathing, also called Belly Breathing, in Chapter 3, but now we will refine the practice with use of the Breath Wave. Working with the Breath Wave teaches you how to control the diaphragm, strengthens your core and entire breathing apparatus, and leads to optimal breathing in your day-to-day activities, including

BREATHE HOW YOU WANT TO FEEL

exercise. The Breath Wave underpins any correcting measures to dysfunctional mechanics in our breathing.†††

The Breath Wave is a foundational breathing technique in yoga and pranayama practices. It's sometimes called the three-part yogic breath or *dirgha pranayama*. Its purpose is to promote deep, conscious breathing, increasing the flow of vital energy in the body and giving you control over the breath. By consciously engaging in rhythmic, deep inhalations and exhalations, you activate the full capacity of your lungs. The Breath Wave technique helps to maintain or increase your lung capacity, and there is good reason to increase your lung capacity.

As we get older, we slowly lose our lung capacity. By age 80, we'll have on average 30 percent less lung capacity than we did in our late teens. And the size of your lungs is an accurate marker how long and healthily you will live. In the 1980s, scientists from the Framingham Study, a 70-year project on heart disease, investigated the link between lung size and lifespan. Analyzing data from 5,200 people, they revealed an unexpected result: the most significant factor in longevity wasn't genetics, nutrition, or how much you exercised—it was lung capacity.[8]

I learned the Breath Wave during my pranayama training decades ago in India and Nepal and use it regularly to this day. The Breath Wave is practiced seated, lying down with the knees bent and falling toward each other, or even walking. If you are just beginning with the practice, I suggest lying down on the floor to offer more support as well as sensorial feedback in the sacrum and back ribs.

---

††† Everly and Lating, "Voluntary Control of Respiration Patterns" in *A Clinical Guide to the Treatment of the Human Stress Response* (New York: Springer, 2019), state, "controlled diaphragmatic breathing stands out as one of the most effective techniques for reducing excessive stress. The researchers concluded that clinicians treating patients experiencing excessive stress syndromes should seriously consider controlled respiration as a suitable intervention for virtually all patients."

For additional somatic feedback, it is helpful to place your hands (or a book) on your belly and sternum.

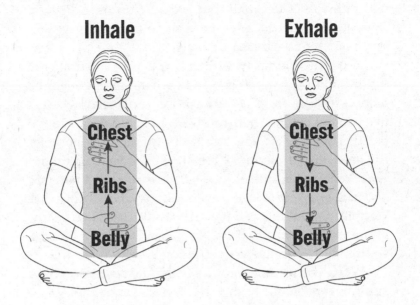

The practice of the Breath Wave involves breathing nasally about 60 percent into the belly, pausing, then about 30 percent breath into the ribs, pausing, breathing the last 10 percent into the clavicle area, and pausing once more.

On the exhale you reverse the wave, breathe out 10 percent from the chest and pause, exhale 30 percent from the ribs and pause, and then complete your exhale as the belly draws slightly inward.

The percentages are approximate, but there will be a sense that you breathe in greater volume lower in the torso. On the inhale, the breath wave moves upward and expands the ribs outward, and on the exhale, there is the descending feeling and sense of downward gravitational pull. Experiment with the percentages and speed of the

Breath Wave to find your own rhythm. You might pause momentarily or even for a few seconds. You can also remove the pauses and just breathe like a wave into the belly, ribs, and chest, and then exhale in reverse. Using a slow, steady cadence tends to calm your nervous system, and a quicker pace increases energy.

Allow the Breath Wave to fill you with air from the inside out that expands wide and then upward. It might be helpful to sit in front of a mirror for visual feedback, just like you did before when you were assessing what type of breather you are. As you breathe in through the nose, let the pressure and volume of breath expand your circumference. You may see or feel your belly expand like a balloon, and in the back rib area, it may feel like you have wings that are spreading. While the Breath Wave proceeds vertically, filling the belly, ribs, and chest, imagine you are stretching yourself wide even as the progression is upward.

When you breathe into the belly, feel your lower back and ribs expand outward. You'll feel this expansion especially when practicing lying down or with your hands in a claw position around your floating ribs.

As you breathe into the midsection, feel the inner pressure expanding your rib cage outward. If you are lying down, you'll feel the back ribs push into the ground as the breath stretches you from within.

Finally, as you take your full breath in and under your collarbones, rather than having your shoulder rise up to your ears, feel the spreading of your shoulders as if someone is pulling back on your shoulders. Be playful and move your body as the breath waves flows in and through you.

On the exhale, feel the descent, the concentration, and the rooting as your ribs and diaphragm return to their neutral position.

Let's practice the Breath Wave now.

PRACTICE

Breath Wave

- Find a comfortable seated posture with your sit bones firmly grounded, spine comfortably straight, eyes closed, and shoulders relaxed. Or find a suitable prone position and place a pillow under your knees (or bend your knees and place your feet flat on the ground). Wear loose clothing around the waist to ensure your abdomen has full range of movement.

- Take a moment to set your intention, perhaps thinking: *I'm practicing the Breath Wave so that my breathing mechanics improve, and I'll be healthy and spread love in the world.*

- Begin with Breath Awareness, observing your breath moving in and out of the nostrils. Observe a few breaths.

- Place one hand or a book on the lower abdomen and the other hand on your sternum.

- **First Phase—Belly.** As you breathe in through the nose, feel the breath pushing your belly and lower back outward. Stay here, only breathing in and out of the belly. Breathe about 60 percent of a full breath into the belly. As you exhale out the nose, feel your abdomen moving inward. Your upper hand should not be moving.

- Repeat this belly-only breathing for about 5 breaths before moving to the next part.

- **Second Phase—Belly and Ribs.** Just like before, breathe in 60 percent into your belly and pause for a moment, and then breathe 30 percent into the middle torso and pause. Feel the internal pressure and your rib cage open with your upper hand. As you exhale, reverse what you just did. Exhaling 30 percent, let your ribs compress naturally and pause, and then exhale fully as your belly moves inward toward your spine.

- Repeat this belly-rib breathing for 5 breaths before moving to the next part.

- **Third Phase—Belly, Ribs, and Chest.** As you breathe in, keeping it nasal just like before, feel your belly expanding to take in 60 percent of a full breath and pause. Then continue to inhale, feeling the ribs expand with another 30 percent, and pause. Finally, inhale under your collarbones 10 percent to maximum capacity and pause. Feel the pressure of a full breath.

- On the controlled exhalation out the nose, expel your breath in reverse order. First, exhale from your chest and pause, then your ribs and pause, and finally your abdomen and pause.

- Repeat this belly-rib-chest breathing for 5 breaths.

- **Fourth Phase—Full Breath Wave.** And now do the full Breath Wave without the pauses 10 times. As you inhale slowly through the nose, feel your belly and back ribs expand, your rib basket opening, and your chest filling up. And then exhale out of your chest, ribs, and belly. Keep your hands on your belly and sternum and feel the ebb and flow of the Breath Wave. Breathing slowly tends to balance your nervous system, and breathing more quickly will bring more energy into your system.

- At the conclusion, let go of trying to breathe in any particular way and let the breath return to its normal rhythm. Rest for a few minutes without the need to do anything at all.

Dedicated practice sessions like the one above where you are seated or lying down are an excellent way to feel the Breath Wave with its nuances and subtleties. It also offers you a conducive environment to cultivate interoceptive awareness and learn how to incorporate the Breath Wave into your breathing tool kit. Eventually, we are endeavoring to unconsciously breathe in the wave-like pattern. For day-to-day breathing, that means the ebb and flow of the wave is slow and remains relatively low in the torso; other times when you are exercising, the wave will be more energetic, filling the abdomen and the chest with the full beautiful wave-like motion.

After you are familiar with a seated practice of the Breath Wave, I encourage you to try it in different positions, which includes standing or during movement such as yoga or tai chi. For example, when I am cycling and hunched over for many hours at a time, there is pressure on the front ribs and diaphragm that restricts movement. I still use the Breath Wave to push the breath into my back and under my scapula; this has stopped feelings of breathlessness and an inability to take a deep breath. When I am in a twisted yoga posture, I use the Breath Wave to protect my back by stabilizing my spine and then expanding and contracting the soft tissue with the movement itself, as if I'm massaging my internal organs. I encourage you to play with the Breath Wave in different bodily positions, such as when exercising, seated in a car or at the computer, walking, and before bed.

Should you be breathing all day using the full Breath Wave? Of course not. While the Breath Wave is a beneficial practice for promoting deep, conscious breathing, it is not necessary or recommended to practice it all day long. Techniques like this three-part Breath Wave are best practiced in dedicated sessions 5 to 20 minutes in length to improve fundamental breathing mechanics and lung capacity. I know many people who use a faster-paced version of the Breath Wave as their morning wake-up practice or before a workout. If it is practiced with a slower pace and slightly less volume of breaths, blood pressure and heart rate is reduced, inducing a state of relaxation and calm. In both cases, you are gaining the short-term benefit of dialing your nervous system to the state you want to feel, and longer-term benefits of training in optimal mechanics.

Below is a Breath Wave practice that incorporates a visualization practice.

PRACTICE

Breath Wave Visualization for Peace and Tranquility

- Find a quiet and comfortable place to sit or lie down. Close your eyes and begin to bring your attention to your breath. Take a moment to relax your body, allowing any tension to melt away.

- Take a moment to set your intention, perhaps thinking: *I'm practicing the Breath Wave to spread peace and tranquility to my family and community.*

- Let's begin the Breath Wave Visualization for Peace.

- Take a slow and light breath in through your nose, filling your abdomen and ribs from the bottom up. Feel your ribs expand in front, on the side, and behind you as you slowly inhale.

- Exhale through the nose and let the breath go.

- Now, as you inhale, imagine a gentle wave of positive energy welling within you, bringing with it a sense of rejuvenation. Visualize this wave as a beautiful, soothing color that resonates with peace.

- As the wave reaches the peak of your inhalation, feel the energy and vitality within your being filling every cell of your body. Pause your breath at the top for a moment. Embrace the uplifting and energizing qualities of this wave. Smile and relax your face.

- Now, exhale slowly through the nose, letting go of any control. Your breath expands outward toward the horizon, touching all beings near and far. Visualize the gentle, colorful wave of breath expanding into relaxed spaciousness. Let any tension or worries drift away.

- Continue this slow-breathing pattern through the nose.

- Inhale a wave of energy toward you, and exhale it outward toward all beings.

- With each breath, feel the replenishing energy filling your body.

- With each slow exhale, feel a sense of spaciousness and deep relaxation spreading throughout your entire being and into the world.

- Let go into to the natural ebb and flow of the breath, finding solace in the gentle rise and fall of the breath wave.

- Stay with this visualization for a few more minutes, fully immersing yourself in the peaceful energy and movement of the breath wave.

- Feel the flow and harmony within you, connecting with the spacious essence of your being.

- When you are ready, let go of the visualization and trying to breathe in any particular way. Let the breath come and go as it likes. Allow the breath to breathe you.

- Wiggle your fingers and toes, stretch your body if that feels good, and open your eyes.

KEY INSIGHTS

- Identifying and correcting any dysfunction in breathing empowers you to live a more resilient, vibrant, and fulfilled life. Most of us have some degree of dysfunctional breathing due to various factors such as stress, poor mechanical habits, and age.

- The nose was designed for breathing, the mouth for eating. The negative consequences of chronic mouth breathing have serious implications for both your physical and mental health in the short and long run.

- Use the Breath Wave's diaphragmatic breathing to train your body to breathe optimally.

Chapter 8

BREATHING FOR
DAILY LIFE

By this time, you know how to use breathing to turn the dials on your nervous system in a conscious and directed manner. You can change your state within a few conscious breaths, whether that is a few physiological sighs, the Conscious Pause, or more extended breathing interventions. You have the know-how and experience to act immediately to change your state.

But the way that we *unconsciously* breathe day-to-day has the most significant impact overall on your sense of well-being than do breathing interventions. We don't want to live our life continually obsessing over what breathing intervention to employ. Of course, life happens, and it isn't always peaceful. So, when stress arises, we intervene at those times appropriately—relying on our breathing tool kit. But ideally, the default way we breathe is optimal, our mechanics are dialed, our blood chemistry is regulated, and we need not interfere too often.

So, how should our breathing be in daily life?

You won't be surprised that optimal day-to-day breathing involves using the nose, breathing low using the diaphragm instead of the upper-chest muscles, and breathing slowly so we don't overbreathe, all done with our tongue and head positioned correctly. In this chapter, we are going to look more closely at how to breathe lightly, low, and slow.

Before we unpack breathing lightly through the nose, let's briefly review some fundamentals.

Nasal breathing is optimal because our paranasal passage is a natural filter, humidifier, and regulator of air temperature. You utilize the nitric oxide that is produced in the sinuses when breathing through the nose, and this helps maximize the oxygen uptake in the lungs. When physical demands are such that you need to breathe with the mouth, you have that option, like when you are carrying heavy groceries upstairs, hiking or running uphill, or dancing energetically. But breathing through the nose in nearly all your daily activities is optimal because it slows down your breathing. Slowing down the breath and reducing the respiratory rate helps improve the efficiency of breathing. By taking slower breaths, you enhance oxygen uptake from the blood and improve overall oxygen delivery to the body's tissues.[1,‡‡‡]

When you breathe through your nose, there is a natural tendency to draw the air low into the lungs with the diaphragm muscle rather than using your upper chest and neck. Breathing low, expanding outwardly, fills the lower lobes of the lungs, where the highest concentration of the alveoli are located and blood gas exchange happens. This allows the lungs to fully expand, which facilitates the optimal exchange of oxygen and carbon dioxide.

---

‡‡‡ This study found that two minutes of slow breathing can reduce sympathetic activity and restore autonomic balance, restore respiratory balance, and reduce blood pressure. The more time you practice per week, the greater the blood pressure reduction.

If, on the other hand, you only breathe into the upper chest, it is not only an inefficient way to move oxygen and carbon dioxide in and out of your system, it also tells your brain that there is a threat nearby, so your fight-or-flight system engages, and stress hormones infuse your system when they're not needed.

The Importance of Increasing Your Tolerance to Carbon Dioxide

Ensuring that you breathe nasally, low, and slow throughout your day reduces or eliminates chronic over-breathing and improves the body's tolerance to carbon dioxide. Why do we want to increase our tolerance to carbon dioxide? If you recall from Respiration 101, hemoglobin in your blood releases oxygen when in the presence of carbon dioxide. With a higher presence of carbon dioxide, oxygen releases into your cells and tissues more readily.

The reason we want to increase our tolerance of carbon dioxide is because our brain, organs, and entire physical body receive more fuel! And consistently breathing through the nose, slowly and using the diaphragm, gradually increases our tolerance to carbon dioxide. As James Nestor wrote succinctly in *Breath*, "What our bodies really want, what they require to function properly, isn't faster or deeper breaths. It's not more air. What we need is more carbon dioxide."

To increase your carbon dioxide tolerance, you can train during your day-to-day activity. When you are moving to and from your home, vacuuming, yardwork, dancing, or even speaking, try to keep your breathing low and slow through the nose. It takes practice. Even when that feeling of breathlessness comes on (because of the slight increase of carbon dioxide in your system from metabolic increase), instead of automatically mouth breathing, breathe slow and low. If you need to take that one big breath through the mouth, that is fine. Then return to low and slow nasal breathing. Draw the breath long and slow into the nose and feel the satisfaction of the breath wave. It takes a little mindfulness to stick with it, and you may feel a slight physical discomfort, but the benefits of the daily training are worth it! Build slowly, breath by breath.

You can also set aside five minutes each day to train in increasing your tolerance to carbon dioxide with the Breathe Light exercise, a practice developed by Patrick McKeown of the Oxygen Advantage. You need not be a professional athlete or elite performer, though those individuals too benefit from the Breathe Light practice. If you practice the Breathe Light exercise consistently twice a day, you'll see your BOLT score notch up a few seconds per week—this has been the case with every individual I have worked with. You'll see a reduction in day-to-day breathlessness and overall downregulation of felt stress and anxiety.

I use the Breathe Light exercise before I meditate because it creates an ideal chemical environment within my body for relaxed concentration and sets a baseline of mental resilience throughout the day. I also Breathe Light for a few minutes right before I speak publicly to reduce anxiety and increase focus. Breathe Light is suitable for everyone, except individuals with panic disorders or when pregnant.

Breathing Lightly

During the Breathe Light exercise, you intentionally reduce the amount of air you breathe, creating a gentle sense of air hunger—that feeling like you'd like to take a deep breath, but you don't. Air hunger indicates that carbon dioxide has accumulated in the blood, which prompts the release of oxygen. By practicing gentle, light, and soft breathing in the Breathe Light exercise, your blood vessels open up, and more oxygen is delivered to your tissues and organs—you actually feel this happening in your body. Breathing lightly and slowly through the nose also takes advantage of nitric oxide in the nasal cavity, purifying the air and opening the airways and blood vessels in the lungs.

Throughout the 4- to 5-minute Breathe Light exercise, it's important to focus on achieving a consistent feeling of air hunger during both inhalation and exhalation. When you feel the urge to take a big breath, relax and stick with the practice, even though you'll feel outside your comfort zone.

While it's not necessary to overly concern yourself with diaphragmatic breathing, if you are already doing so, that's good. The primary focus during this exercise is on progressively slowing down the breath, making it quieter, and softening its intensity, breathing in 50 to 70 percent of your normal inhale. The goal of this practice is altering your internal chemistry. You'll feel that through the sensation of air hunger, which should remain manageable.

If the air hunger becomes too strong, let go of the exercise for a few breaths, allow yourself to reset, and then resume. As you reduce your breathing volume, you may experience slight tension in your diaphragm muscle, which is normal. However, if you notice involuntary contractions of the diaphragm, it means the air hunger is too intense. The aim is to maintain a tolerable air hunger for around four minutes—find your edge and stay there.

If your breathing rhythm becomes fast or irregular, it means the air hunger is excessive or that you reduced the volume too quickly. In such cases, stop the exercise, breathe normally for 30 seconds, and then resume gentle, light breathing to reestablish a tolerable level of air hunger. Avoid intentionally interfering with your breathing muscles or holding your breath. Instead, allow your breath to soften through relaxation, taking slow and gentle nasal breaths.

PRACTICE

Breathe Light

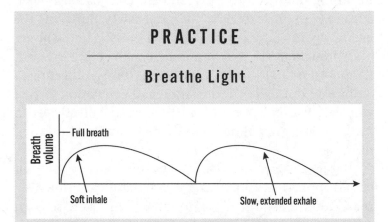

- Find a comfortable position, seated or lying down. Lean back if it is comfortable but keep your back upright and relaxed.

- Set your intention, perhaps by thinking: *May my Breathe Light practice benefit my body and mind so that I can be of service to my family and community.*

- Turn your attention to your breath and observe it without changing anything. This is breath awareness. Notice the cooler air moving into your nostrils and the slightly warmer air exiting.

- Relax your face, your shoulders, and your belly.

- Begin your Breathe Light practice by progressively reducing the speed of each breath as it comes into and out of your nose.

- Breathe very lightly. Slow down your breathing such that you barely feel the air moving in and out of your nostrils.

- Breathe so tranquil and serene that the delicate hairs inside your nostrils remain still, undisturbed by the airflow.

- Progressively reduce the amount of air you breathe in to be around 50 to 70 percent of a normal breath, until you feel like you'd like to breathe in more air.

- You are creating a tolerable air hunger, and this is good.

- Find that sensation of air hunger and relax into it, even though you feel like taking a larger breath. Go easy, and find your edge.

- If the feeling is too strong, you are feeling stressed, or you lose control of your breathing, take a break for 30 seconds, relax, breathe normally, and then start again.

- It's no problem to take a rest.

- Continue to practice the Breathe Light for about 5 minutes.

- At the conclusion, let go of the Breathe Light practice, rest silently, and observe how you feel in your body and in mind.

- Repeat 2 or 3 times a day, including before going to sleep.

Unconscious Breath Holding

In Chapter 5, we explored the remarkable power of conscious breath holding. It serves as a pattern interrupter, enhancing our resiliency to stress, regulating our energy levels, and strengthening our lung capacity and carbon dioxide tolerance. Conscious breath holding is a gift that keeps on giving!

Unconscious breath holding, on the other hand, has many negative consequences. We often hold our breath unconsciously when we brace ourselves against external stressors. Watch family members during an argument cross their arms over their chest and stop breathing, ready to explode. When traffic on the freeway is frantic or even when a stoplight seems to stay red for too long, often we hold our breath because of fear or frustration. Even opening the bills in the mail, hearing a helicopter overhead, or watching the news causes some of us to brace against uncertainty, stopping our breathing. External stressors are innumerable and merge with our unique character, often resulting in unconscious breath holding.

One modern circumstance affects a majority of us that leads to unconscious breath holding. Research reveals that as much as 75 percent of Americans unconsciously hold their breath while responding to e-mails, texting, or scrolling.[§§§] This phenomenon has been labeled *e-mail apnea*, *screen apnea*, or *scrolling apnea* and is characterized by shallow, upper-chest breathing and frequent, unconscious breath holding during digital interactions. *Apnea* is a Greek word; *a* means "not" and *pnea* refers to breathing—literally meaning "without breath." With the average

---

[§§§] Linda Stone coined the term *e-mail apnea* in 2008. And the first published research was Lin and Peper, "Psychophysiological Patterns During Cell Phone Text Messaging: A Preliminary Study," *Applied Psychophysiology and Biofeedback* 34z no. 1 (March 2009): 53–57, doi: 10.1007/s10484-009-9078-1.

American spending over seven hours a day in front of screens, consider how much breathless, stress-inducing time is accumulated.

Whether it's e-mail apnea or for other reasons, unconsciously holding our breath often turns up our sympathetic nervous system. Our bodies perceive danger as we experience sensations somewhere between breathlessness and suffocation. Blood oxygen saturation levels can drop dangerously, causing pulses of adrenaline and other stress hormones to prepare for fight-or-flight responses. Often, we only become aware of our breath holding when startled by a gasp reflex, followed by a racing heartbeat and symptoms like tinnitus. If left unaddressed, chronic unconscious breath holding has dire effects on our mental and physical health.

So, what is the antidote to unconscious breath holding throughout the day? AIR—awareness, intervention, and regulation. It begins with the first tool in your breathing tool kit: awareness.

When you notice that you've been unconsciously holding your breath, resume breathing and then take a moment to reflect on the preceding situation. Was it a thought, emotion, or mental stressor that provoked the breath holding? Was it something in your physical surroundings, a person, or a specific situation? Perhaps keep a journal or a list of the times you notice. Becoming aware of these stressors empowers you to regain control over your reactions and emotions. Remember, we reclaim our power when we recognize the space between stimulation and response! In that space, you initiate a breathing intervention that downregulates your nervous system. It can be as simple as an extended exhale.

It may also be helpful to plan for situations that typically elicit your unconscious breath holding. Before opening your bank statement, sitting in the waiting room at the doctor's office, or scrolling through your social media news feed—whatever scenarios that tend to induce that nervous state leading to your breath holding—try this straightforward pattern interrupt:

- Place your hand on your belly.

- Inhale and feel your belly expanding into your hand.

- Exhale and slightly press in for feedback.

- Do that two more times.

- Think to yourself: *I am consciously moving into this situation that sometimes causes stress. I'm safe. I'm confident. Empowered with my breath, I'll proceed.*

- And continue.

KEY INSIGHTS

- While breathing interventions are excellent ways to change your state in real time, your everyday breathing is key to your holistic well-being. Your default breathing should be through the nose, low, and slow.

- Increasing tolerance to carbon dioxide enhances oxygen delivery to your brain and organs, improving overall health and making you more resilient to stress. Use the Breathe Light exercise daily to increase your tolerance to carbon dioxide and promote relaxation, concentration, and recovery.

- Many of us unconsciously hold our breath, including when scrolling on our phones, on the computer, or when we are stressed. Unconscious breath holding adversely affects our health. To counter this habit, it's essential to develop interoception and apply appropriate breathing interventions.

Chapter 9

BREATHING FOR SLEEP

The impact of sleep quality on our overall well-being cannot be overstated. Adequate sleep is essential for the rejuvenation and restoration of our bodies. Consistently having seven to eight hours of restful sleep each night is associated with numerous health advantages, including a strengthened immune system, improved cardiovascular health, and a decreased likelihood of developing chronic ailments. Deep sleep is pivotal, no matter our age, for consolidating memories, facilitating learning, and regulating our emotions. Gone are the days when functioning on four or five hours of sleep a night is considered a strength. Prioritizing and maintaining a healthy sleep routine is crucial for optimizing our mental and physical health.[1]

Insufficient sleep quality has a range of short-term repercussions on both our physical and mental health, including daytime fatigue, resulting in diminished alertness and brain fog. Energy levels are compromised, making it a challenge to concentrate and stay focused on our children, school, or work, and it contributes to sexual dysfunction. Cognitive functions, including memory, decision making, and problem solving, are negatively affected. The emotional toll is evident as well, with increased irritability, mood swings, and a sense of emotional instability that strains relationships with our loved ones.

Persistent inadequate sleep has been associated with a heightened risk of chronic conditions such cancer, Alzheimer's, depression, anxiety, obesity, stroke, chronic pain, diabetes, and heart attacks. As the neuroscientist Matthew Walker writes in *Why We Sleep: Unlocking the Power of Sleep and Dreams,* "there does not seem to be one major organ within the body, or process within the brain, that is not optimally enhanced by sleep (and detrimentally impaired when we don't get enough)." In fact, the leading causes of disease and death in developed nations, including heart disease, obesity, dementia, diabetes, and cancer, according to Dr. Walker, all have recognized, causal links to lack of sleep.[2]

So what role does breathing have in our sleep quality? It has a huge role!

Your breathing patterns and habits during the day have a direct impact on how you breathe while you sleep, ultimately influencing the quality of your sleep. The way you breathe during wakefulness sets the foundation for your breathing during sleep. If you have healthy, optimal breathing habits during the day, it is more likely that you will maintain those habits during sleep.

Ensuring nasal breathing during the day and night is the most crucial modification you can make to optimize your sleep quality. Persistent mouth breathing throughout the day almost guarantees its continuation during sleep, producing a series of adverse consequences. Mouth breathing leads to snoring and obstructive sleep apnea, a severe disorder where breathing stops for 10 seconds or more, sometimes occurring as many as 30 times an hour during the night. People often wake up due to snoring, snorting, or gasping for breath, resulting in frequent "micro-awakenings" that disrupt full sleep cycles. At least 25 million American adults suffer from obstructive sleep apnea alone, not to mention the many other sleep disorders, of which many go undiagnosed.[3]

As we mentioned in Part I, mouth breathing bypasses the nose's natural filtration system, permitting easier entry of allergens and pollutants into the airways, potentially aggravating respiratory issues. Mouth breathing also contributes to dehydration, dry mouth, and unpleasant breath since the mouth lacks the moisturizing and purifying effects of nasal breathing. Chronic mouth breathing poses risks to dental health, increasing the likelihood of cavities, gum disease, and misalignment. The imbalance between oxygen and carbon dioxide levels resulting from mouth breathing further disrupts the body's physiological processes and detrimentally impacts sleep. Embracing nasal breathing as a cornerstone of your sleep routine will have profound benefits for your restfulness and overall health.

In addition to nasal breathing throughout the day, the more you develop your breathing tool kit, the better sleep you will have. Sleeping with your mouth closed, resting the tongue on the roof of your mouth, and breathing slowly and diaphragmatically sets you up for restorative sleep. You can help yourself, as mentioned in Chapter 4, by taping your mouth closed (really, I can't recommend it enough!). While it may take a few nights to get used to mouth taping, the multitude of short and long-term advantages make it worthwhile to persevere with this simple practice. The benefits derived from maintaining nasal breathing during sleep far outweigh any minor inconvenience associated with mouth taping.

Basic Routine for Improving Your Sleep

Before we practice a proven breathing technique to prepare you for restorative sleep, below are basic guidelines for your sleep routine. Of course we might not be able to apply all these recommendations, but stacking as many as possible will exponentially benefit you over time.

What to do before sleep:

- **Breathing to Prepare for Sleep:** Before bed, engage in 5 to 15 minutes of conscious breathing that promotes a relaxation response. This includes slow Belly Breathing, where you exhale longer than you inhale, or any other calming breathing patterns recommended in this book, such as the Humming Bee practice or the Breathe Light practice. By slowing your breath and elongating your exhale, you activate the parasympathetic nervous system, signaling your body to relax and prepare for sleep.

- **Mouth Tape:** If you tend to sleep with your mouth open, snore, have nocturnal urination, or wake up with a dry mouth or chapped lips, mouth taping is recommended. Mouth taping is fully explained in Chapter 4.

- **Intention Setting:** Take a moment to set your intention for how you want your mind to be during sleep; some call this programming their subconscious. By consciously directing your thoughts and focusing on positive affirmations or feelings of love and empathy, you create a more conducive mental state for restful sleep.

- **Sleep Schedule**: Aim to establish a consistent sleep schedule by going to bed and waking up at the same time, even after a poor night's sleep or on weekends. This helps regulate your body's internal clock and enhances sleep quality by aligning your natural sleep-wake rhythms.

- **Room Temperature**: Keep your bedroom temperature cool, around 65 degrees Fahrenheit. If your feet tend to get cold, wearing socks helps regulate your overall body temperature and improve comfort during sleep.

- **Insomnia**: If you experience difficulty falling asleep or wake up in the middle of the night and struggle to return to sleep, it's recommended to get out of bed and engage in quiet and relaxing activities. This might include reading, listening to soothing music, or practicing gentle stretching until you feel the urge to sleep again. Avoid screens altogether when rising in the middle of the night, including while in the bathroom. Before getting back in bed, consciously extend your exhales with slow Belly Breathing for a few minutes. Insomnia is a common issue, affecting as many as one in three adults, and it's important to find strategies that work for you.

- **Sunlight:** Exposure to sunlight, especially in the early hours of the day, plays a crucial role in establishing your circadian rhythm by regulating the release of hormones to promote alertness. Sunlight in the morning also creates an internally scheduled release in the evening of melatonin, a hormone that regulates sleep-wake cycles. Spending 10 to 15 minutes outside within the first 20 minutes of waking will help you fall asleep at night.

What to avoid:

- **Extended Eating Window:** Close your eating window at least two hours before bed. Eating a heavy meal one to three hours before bedtime can lead to discomfort and indigestion, making it harder to fall asleep. Your body needs time to digest food properly before lying down, so try to finish your last meal or snack a couple hours before going to sleep.

- **Limit Alcohol:** Stop drinking alcohol a few hours before going to sleep. While alcohol may initially make you feel relaxed and help you fall asleep faster, it disrupts the natural sleep cycles and leads to fragmented and restless sleep.

- **Turn Off Screens:** Avoid all screens at least 90 minutes before bed. The blue light emitted by electronic devices such as smartphones, tablets, and computers suppresses the production of melatonin, the hormone that regulates sleep. Using screens in bed delays the onset of sleep and disrupts the circadian rhythm. It's best to create a technology-free zone in the evening to allow your brain to wind down and prepare for sleep.

- **Tech-Free Bedroom**: Keep the room tech-free, with no computers or televisions. Having electronic devices in the bedroom can be distracting and stimulates the brain, making it harder to relax and fall asleep.

- **Avoid Sleeping on Your Back**: Sleeping on the back is not advised because the position allows your tongue and jaw to slump back and obstruct your airway. The optimal sleep position is lying on either your right or left side. In the yogic tradition, sleeping on the right side is advised because it is said to stimulate the left nostril to be dominant, which promotes rest and relaxation. The Buteyko tradition, on the other hand, advises sleeping on the left side to decrease gastric reflux during sleep and promoting better digestive comfort. Alternatively, sleeping on your belly minimizes overbreathing due to the weight of your body, though there may be strain on the neck or spine.

- **Limit Caffeine**: Avoid caffeine after 1 P.M. Caffeine is a stimulant that interferes with sleep. Even if you feel the immediate effects of caffeine wearing off, it often disrupts your sleep cycle and makes it harder to fall and remain asleep.

- **Exercise During the Day**: Engaging in vigorous exercise close to bedtime may increase alertness through the release of hormones. It stimulates the body, making it challenging to wind down and relax. It's best to schedule exercise earlier in the day,

allowing enough time for your body to
cool down and for your exercise-induced
adrenaline levels to return to normal
before sleep.

Breathing Practices Before Bed

There are many breathing techniques that you can
do before bed, and you need to find the one that works
best for you. Your nervous system might react differently
than mine, so there is not a one-size-fits all practice. That
said, slow breathing with extended exhales often creates
a parasympathetic response, and this is needed for deep
rest. Techniques such as Breathe Light, Humming Bee,
slow Belly Breathing, or Box Breathing are often beneficial
before sleep.

Breath counting methods are also useful and you might
find them particularly effective if you have a racing mind.
There is a special magic in the act of counting your breaths.
Counting is handled by the same area of the brain that's
responsible for worrying. The brain can't count and worry
at the same time, so as Dr. Leah Lagos tells us, "Counting
is exceptionally effective at crowding out stress, calming a
busy brain, and enhancing focus."[4]

Below is a practice of Serenity Breath. It uses a counting with the cadence of 4-7-8. You inhale for a 4 count,
hold for 7, and exhale for an 8 count. You don't have to
inhale to 100 percent capacity and exhale fully. Rather,
slowly inhale for a 4 count (about 75 percent capacity),
feeling your belly and ribs expand, hold your breath while
relaxing your tongue, face, and shoulders, and then slowly
exhale for an 8 count, feeling the bottom of your breath.
By this time, you know to keep it nasal because of the
many benefits over mouth breathing.

The 4-7-8 Serenity Breath is taken from the many Cadence Breathing techniques found in pranayama. Dr. Andrew Weil has taught this 4-7-8 cadence for many years and calls it a "natural tranquilizer for the nervous system." Research has shown that the 4-7-8 technique slows your heart rate and lowers your blood pressure.[5] Dr. Weil suggests inhaling through the nose and exhaling out the mouth with pursed lips, though when practicing the Serenity Breath to induce sleep, exhaling out the nose is recommended. Experiment and find what works best for you.

PRACTICE

Serenity Breath

- Find a comfortable position, lying down on whatever side is most comfortable (but not on your back).

- Before starting the Serenity Breath, set your intention for how you want to sleep through the night, perhaps thinking: *May I drift effortlessly into restorative sleep so that I wake up with energy to spread love in the world.*

- Turn your attention to your breath for a moment and practice breath awareness. No need to change, just notice how you are breathing in this moment.

- Place your tongue comfortably on your upper pallet, slightly behind but not touching your teeth.

- Smile and relax the face.

- Breathe slowly in and out of your nose. Feel the cool air coming into the nostrils and the warm air leaving.

- Then begin your 4-7-8 Serenity Breath cadence.

- Breathe in through the nose softly for a 4 count. Fill to about 75 percent capacity.

- Hold your breath for a 7 count while relaxing the face, shoulders, and neck.

- Exhale slowly through the nose for an 8 count. Feel the bottom of your breath.

- Continue for 5 to 10 rounds (if you drift off, have a restful night!).

- After you finish, let go of the 4-7-8 cadence and rest in that spacious feeling.

- Good night.

KEY INSIGHTS

- Make it a priority to have seven to eight hours of restful sleep for the sake of your overall well-being, brain function, memory health, and emotional balance.

- Keep your mouth closed while you sleep.

- Adopt effective sleep hygiene, including presleep rituals such as consciously down-regulating your nervous system with your breath, a tech-free bedroom, and intention setting. Learn and use the 4-7-8 Serenity Breath practice.

Chapter 10

BREATHING FOR EXERCISE

The way we breathe during exercise is governed by our everyday breathing habits. It is crucial to establish proper breathing mechanics, particularly diaphragmatic and nasal breathing as outlined earlier, in our daily lives if we expect to get the most out of our exercise. If we have poor breathing mechanics or overbreathe most of the day, it will carry over into our one-hour workout, into the gym, or while we are out on the playing field or the bike. This, however, doesn't mean that we shouldn't exercise until we have our breathing mechanics fully optimized. We still work on our breathing during exercise. In this chapter, we are going to look at how breathing interventions before, during, and after exercise help prevent injury, enhance endurance, and promote overall physical well-being.

But before delving into those three key components of this chapter, let's take a moment to recognize the paramount importance of breathing itself during exercise!

We must remember that breathing provides the vital fuel—oxygen—for our muscles and brain. If our breathing patterns are inefficient, this critical fuel supply is compromised. Through personal experience and experimentation, I've come to realize that breathing surpasses sleep, nutrition, and even hydration in its significance. Imagine running or cycling for an hour on poor sleep or not eating or drinking—it's possible. But could you do the same without breathing for even a few minutes? Not a chance. It is evident how crucial the breath is!

Nasal Breathing and Exercise

We have discussed the many benefits of nasal breathing over mouth breathing throughout this book. The same benefits apply while we are exercising. While intense physical demands may necessitate mouth breathing at times, we train ourselves to breathe predominantly through the nose even when our metabolism increases. In doing so, we benefit from:

Increased Oxygen Uptake: Nasal breathing introduces approximately 50 percent more resistance compared to mouth breathing because the nasal passage is smaller than the mouth. This resistance is beneficial because it results in approximately 20 percent more oxygen absorption into our bloodstream. This enhanced oxygen uptake fuels our muscles and optimizes performance.

Moisture Retention: Nasal breathing helps you from becoming dehydrated. Mouth breathing leads to a significant loss of moisture, with 42 percent more water escaping compared to nasal breathing. To experience this firsthand, try breathing onto your mobile phone screen using your nose and then your mouth—observe how much more moisture dissipates from the mouth.

Nitric Oxide Benefits: Breathing through the nose promotes vasodilation and bronchodilation through the diffusion of nitric oxide. This improves blood flow, delivering more oxygen and nutrients to our muscles, while also enhancing respiratory function.

Overbreathing and Exercise

We have also previously explored the detrimental effects—physically and cognitively—of overbreathing. Overbreathing is breathing more than our metabolic demands require. When we exercise, the demands on our physical system often lead to an increase in the strength, pace, and depth of our breaths—all three breathing dials are turned up. While we may need to mouth breathe at times during a steep hill or when our activity intensifies, if we are chronically overbreathing during exercise, the balance in our blood gases are disrupted.

Overbreathing causes us to blow off too much carbon dioxide, leading our bodies to maladapt. As a result of this maladaptation, the delivery of oxygen to our brain and organs is compromised. Rapid upper-chest panting associated with overbreathing during sports or exercise proves inefficient as it fails to make the most of the air in our lungs and hinders the effective delivery of oxygen to our cells. Not only are our muscles impacted, it also results in poor decision-making precisely at the time when we need our A game.

Furthermore, overbreathing and blood gas dysregulation causes imbalances in your electrolytes like sodium, calcium, and potassium. Electrolytes, those key ingredients in all your nutrition and sports drinks, are crucial for cell communication through electrical impulses. An excessively alkaline pH in the blood (from overbreathing) causes electrolytes to shift into muscle and brain cells rather than remaining in the fluid surrounding them. Dehydration leads to muscle spasms, weakness, and fatigue. If you want to stay maximally hydrated, keep it nasal![1]

So, during all physical activity, our aim is to maintain nasal breathing for as much as possible. This is challenging—I know!

Begin training today. When you go to the gym, ride your bike to pick up your child at school, walk briskly to the office, or jog a couple of miles around the neighborhood, keep it nasal. If you become out of breath, rather than mouth breathe, slow down the speed and reduce your exertion, which will allow you to breathe nasally. This takes training. In this way, you'll begin to adapt your system to tolerate a higher concentration of carbon dioxide, which ensures the most efficient delivery of oxygen to your cells, promoting enhanced physical and cognitive performance and increasing your lung capacity, all of which contribute to a longer health span. Health span is, according to Dr. Peter Attia, the period of our life spent in good health, free from chronic diseases and disabilities of aging. Health span emphasizes not only the length of one's life but also the quality of life during those years. In other words, health span focuses on maintaining well-being and function as opposed to simply extending your lifespan. And nasal breathing is key to a long health span.

Breathing Efficiency, Exercise Economy, and Making Better Decisions

The relationship between your heart rate, respiratory rate, and energy consumption is closely intertwined. When you breathe faster, your heart beats faster, and more energy is expended in the process of respiration. While aerobic training is commonly focused on improving muscular performance, it's equally important to train our respiratory system for enhanced breathing efficiency, exercise economy, and brain function. This is why we breathe through our nose—it is more efficient.

By breathing slower through your nose even while exercising, you significantly improve oxygen uptake in your tissues. As you reduce your respiratory rate, your heartbeat also slows down, even when your intensity increases. This signifies your growing efficiency in extracting oxygen from each breath and effectively transferring it to the muscles. This means that you expend less energy on breathing, which allows more energy to be available for the actual work performed by your muscles and brain. In essence, as you enhance your breathing efficiency by breathing less, you unlock a greater reserve of energy for the physical activity you engage in. By optimizing your respiratory system, you maximize your overall physical performance and enjoyment.

An important but often overlooked benefit of nasal breathing during exercise is enhanced executive function and motor skills. This especially matters when you need it most, like when you're making quick decisions (turning fast on skis, snowboard, or a mountain bike). Or in team sports when you're playmaking in midfield or passing on a fast break while running down the basketball court.

Additionally, enhanced cognitive skills help prevent injuries in the gym when technique is critical to safe resistance training.

Fire Up Your System Before Exercise

Just as you warm up and stretch your muscles before exercising, it is recommended to do the same for your respiratory muscles. The diaphragm is the most important muscle involved in breathing, along with the intercostals, and a proper warm-up allows them to fully contribute to efficient breathing and fueling of your system. By massaging, stretching, and warming up your diaphragm and intercostals, you'll not only enhance their flexibility and reduce the risk of strain or injury but also improve their overall function.

Any of the upregulating breathing interventions that we have discussed earlier can be used as preparation before exercise, training, or competition. I encourage you to find one that works with the amount of time you have, and use a few minutes of self-massage or gentle rolling of the diaphragm, intercostals, and middle and upper back. If you are prone to anxiety before competition, be sure not to dial your system too high before the event!

The Diaphragm Warm-Up Exercise below is a perfect preparation. By incorporating respiratory warm-up exercises like this, you'll enhance your breathing capacity and optimize your overall performance. The Diaphragm Warm-Up Exercise has three rounds of diaphragmatic breathing with breath holds. Each round is slightly different. In round 1, you hold your breath after exhaling (pyramid breath). In round 2, you hold after inhaling (inverted pyramid breath). And in round 3, you hold your breath after both inhaling and exhaling (Box Breathing). The breath count in the practice below is 5, but you can adjust accordingly. In between each round, you take 10 deep nasal breaths. There are 45 breaths in the Diaphragm Warm-Up Exercise, and it should take 5 to 10 minutes.

PRACTICE

Diaphragm Warm-Up Exercise

Find a comfortable position, seated or lying down. For a few minutes, use your fingertips to massage the edge and underneath your rib cage, from your sternum around to your back ribs. Rub your intercostals in between the rib bones. Breathe slow and long while you massage.

Then, set your intention, perhaps thinking: *May my breathing practice connect my body and mind, prepare me, and strengthen me as I move through the world to spread joy.*

Then, drop into stillness. Close your eyes. Feel your body. Hover your attention over and around the body and just notice.

Shift your attention to notice how you feel emotionally. Just notice.

Then, turn your attention to your breath and take a few moments to feel the movement in and out of the nostrils. If you like, place your hand on your belly and sternum or around your rib basket.

ROUND 1: PYRAMID BREATH

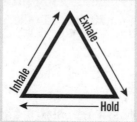

Inhale for a 5 count, expanding the belly and ribs to 75 percent capacity.

Exhale for a 5 count, releasing and letting go.

Hold after your exhale for a 5 count.

Repeat 4 more times.

Then, take 10 slow diaphragmatic breaths through the nose.

ROUND 2: INVERTED PYRAMID BREATH

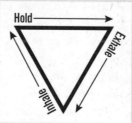

Inhale for a 5 count, expanding the belly and ribs to 75 percent capacity or more.

Hold with a full breath for a 5 count.

Exhale for a 5 count, releasing and letting go.

Repeat 4 more times.

Then, take 10 diaphragmatic breaths through the nose, increasing the pace from Round 1.

ROUND 3: BOX BREATHING

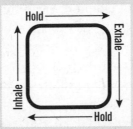

Inhale for a 5 count, expanding the belly and ribs to near capacity.

Hold with a full breath for a 5 count. Relax.

Exhale for a 5 count, releasing and letting go.

Hold after you exhale for a 5 count.

Repeat 4 more times.

Take 10 deep, diaphragmatic breaths through the nose, increasing the pace from Round 2.

After your final breath, exhale and hold your breath.

Watch. Dwell within.

When you feel the need to breathe, let your breath come back naturally.

Rest for a few moments and notice how you feel in your body and mind.

Breathing During Exercise

For the last few years, I've competed in long-distance multiday self-supported mountain bike races. The courses are in remote and extreme terrain, and we cycle 15 to 20 hours a day multiple days in a row. While my preparation incorporated the usual strength and endurance training regimen of an endurance cyclist, the most impactful element to my performance has been breath training.

The breath training that I'm referring to is what we are discussing in this chapter: warming up the diaphragm and intercostal properly, using the exercise intensity dial that we'll discuss below, and breathing for recovery. If I neglected any aspect of this, fuel for my engine was lacking.

I'm not a professional athlete by any measure. I'm a recreational athlete. But using the breath for performance is beneficial, whether you're an elite athlete or a weekend warrior because it allows us to maximize our stamina and strength, enhance our mental focus and concentration, and above all, enjoy moving our bodies. I take inspiration from observing the likes of breath-conscious athletes like LeBron James, Roger Federer, Gerry Lopez, Laird Hamilton, Mary Decker, and Sanya Richards-Ross. Honed awareness, extending exhales to gain respiratory control, and regulating breath during intense competition are the pivotal components that underlie their success.

Exercise Intensity Dial

Expanding upon Chapter 3's breathing dials of strength, pace, and depth, we now introduce a new dial: the exercise intensity dial (EID). The EID serves as a practical tool to help us monitor and adjust our breathing patterns in real time, using nasal and mouth breathing when appropriate. The EID integrates mindfulness, interoception, and a combination of nasal and mouth breathing techniques at different intensities. Its purpose is to not only enhance our performance and endurance but also counteract the negative effects of improper breathing patterns that contribute to fatigue.

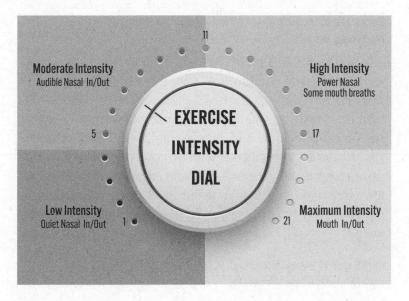

Moderate Intensity
Audible Nasal In/Out

High Intensity
Power Nasal
Some mouth breaths

EXERCISE INTENSITY DIAL

11

5

17

Low Intensity
Quiet Nasal In/Out   1

Maximum Intensity
Mouth In/Out

21

The EID is described below. Keep in mind that everyone has unique physical and respiratory fitness levels. Make adjustments according to your needs, progressively dialing up as your intensity increases and dialing back down as you regain control of your breath.

Clicks 1 to 4: Quiet Nasal In/Out—Low Intensity—Balanced Breath

Use clicks 1 to 4, the lower end of the EID, for low-intensity activities such as yoga, Pilates, golf, or warming up on a bike or rower. This is nasal breathing that offers you enhanced filtration, warming, and humidification of the air. Additionally, nasal breathing promotes increased production and inhalation of nitric oxide, a vasodilator and bronchodilator. Nasal breathing importantly maintains the optimal blood gas balance and proper uptake of oxygen into your muscles.

Clicks 5 to 10: Audible Nasal In/Out—Moderate Intensity—Increasing Breath

Dial to clicks 5 to 10 during moderate-intensity activity like jogging, swimming, dancing, or jumping rope. This corresponds to higher aerobic activity where you can still speak normally but require additional breaths. By focusing on slow and deep nasal inhales and exhales, you stimulate the engagement of your diaphragm, optimize oxygen uptake into cells, and improve carbon dioxide exchange. This deliberate approach to breathing helps regulate your breathing rate, leading to enhanced endurance and overall performance physically and cognitively.

Clicks 11 to 17: Power Nasal In/Nasal Out or Nasal in/Mouth Out—High Intensity—Intense Breath

Clicks 11 to 17 is the transitional stage where nasal breathing remains the primary focus, albeit with increased challenges. Speaking becomes less possible because of the intensity of the activity. You may need to powerfully inhale and exhale through the nose. Or you might need to switch to inhaling through the nose and exhaling out the mouth for a few breaths, blowing off carbon dioxide, which temporarily alleviates breathlessness, and then return to nasal only. Maintaining nasal breathing as much as possible is encouraged, even if occasional mouth exhales occur. It's a challenge to stay nasal only with these higher-intensity activities, such as powerful paddling, energetic Zumba classes or dancing, cycling or running up a hill, or intense spinning sessions. This demands your attention. Try not to revert to panting continually through the mouth.

Clicks 18 to 21: Mouth In/Mouth Out—Maximum Intensity—Power Breath

When exercising at maximal exertion, your EID is turned all the way up. This is for activities such as hill sprints, tabata sessions, circuit training, or high-intensity interval training (HIIT) workouts. During maximum-intensity efforts, mouth breathing becomes necessary to facilitate greater airflow, oxygen supply, and blowing off excessive carbon dioxide. However, try to turn the dial down a few clicks as soon as the intensity lessens, as nasal breathing offers more physiological advantages and quickens recovery in the short and long terms. Dialing down to nasal breathing should be prioritized whenever possible, turning your EID from mouth in/out, to nose in/mouth out, to nasal only.

Remember, the goal is to dial your breathing appropriate to the intensity of your exercise, gradually moving up or down one click at a time. Proceed click by click. Like when you are driving a manual stick shift car, move up and down through the gears one after another, not jumping too quickly.

Training with this EID system in mind, you optimize your breathing patterns to enhance physical performance and mental clarity, increase endurance, and recover optimally. Eventually, the EID becomes internalized, and your body and breath know how and when to turn the dial up and down, depending on the intensity of your activity.

Breathing for Recovery

There has been a significant increase in the study of recovery for athletes over the last decade.[2] This trend is not limited to professional athletes alone; even those of us who exercise primarily for our health and enjoyment have benefited from the advancements in sports science and the growing recognition of the significance of recovery.

This broader perspective acknowledges that recovery plays a crucial role in adaptation, repair, and extending our health span.

Why is recovery so important?

Exercise, especially higher intensities, is an acute stressor on the body and mind. The physiological processes triggered during exercise are catabolic, meaning that they break muscle down to use the body's energy for fuel and activation. We need recovery to restore, adapt, and become stronger. As Dr. Epel writes, "Your body loves acute stress. This process of peak and recovery—of sympathetic nervous system action followed by parasympathetic nervous system action, triggering cell cleanup and repair—is wonderful for us. In fact, we need it."[3]

What this means is that we get fitter and stronger during recovery, not during exercise! Strenuous exercises and strength training taxes and depletes our system, breaking it down. Exercise sets off the release of stress hormones like adrenaline and cortisol and other inflammatory markers. The postexercise period is when we want to move toward parasympathetic dominance, downshifting to allow our muscles and systems to adapt and recover. To ensure effective adaptation to the stress of exercise, we must downregulate and focus on recovery right after our workouts or training sessions.

After completing a workout or physical activity, it's common to neglect this crucial step of transitioning our bodies into recovery mode. If we fail to initiate the recovery process immediately, we risk carrying those elevated stress levels with us throughout the day, affecting our interactions at work, causing us to drive through traffic in an agitated manner, or meaning we spend time at home with family while stressed out. To fully reap the benefits of our physical exertion, prioritizing postexercise recovery is essential, and it can be jump-started even before leaving the gym or reaching for our phones to check social media.[4] Devoting five minutes or longer after exercise to restorative breathing techniques releases acetylcholine that not only calms your organs but also stimulates your body's release of serotonin, dopamine, and prolactin, those feel-good hormones.[5]

Here are two standard breathing interventions to jump-start your recovery.

4:6 Breathing Cadence: Focus on slow, nasal-only diaphragmatic breathing. Extend your exhales to find a 4:6 count; inhaling for a 4 count and exhaling for a 6 count. Extended exhalations while counting induces rest and recovery. Simple and effective.

Tactile Breathing: Place your thumbs and fingers around your lower ribs. Feel the expansion of the belly and lower ribs on the inhale and the contraction of them on the exhale. Inhale and exhale slowly through the nose, extending your exhale longer than your inhale. Use whatever cadence works for you, making sure you exhale longer than you inhale. Activate your rest-and-digest response in your nervous system with Tactile Breathing.

So-Hum Mantra for Recovery

Another potent technique for recovery is the use of the So-Hum mantra. While it may initially seem peculiar to include a mantra in the context of exercise, I have observed the effectiveness of this practice firsthand in myself and in others. I can attest that mentally or quietly reciting these two syllables, "sooooo" and "huummm," synchronized with the inhalation and exhalation, has proven to be remarkably beneficial in aiding recovery following intense physical exertion, alleviating exercise-induced asthma symptoms, calming an overactive mind, and activating the relaxation response after prolonged physical and mental efforts. Studies have shown how mantra-based meditations—like the So-Hum practices—slow the heart rate, reduce blood pressure, increase heart rate variability, and decrease breathing rate, all of which contribute to recovery from stress of exercise or otherwise.[6]

So-Hum is a foundational mantra of pranayama. The mantra encapsulates the very essence of the inhalation and exhalation sounds, and has other related esoteric explanations. The technique itself is straightforward. During the inhalation, you mentally or quietly recite "soooooooooo." On the exhalation, "huuuuuuummmmm" is quietly voiced with lips closed or mentally recited. If you need to catch your breath after exercise or are experiencing an elevated respiratory rate due to external stressors, practice So-Hum and attentively listen and feel the resonating vibrations of the sound emanating within your skull, feeling the cranial resonance in the center of your head.

By incorporating the So-Hum mantra into our recovery routine, we tap in to the harmonizing power of the breath and facilitate relaxation. Its simplicity, combined with its ability to regulate and calm the breath, makes it an invaluable tool in promoting recovery, interrupting negative thought loops, and fostering a state of inner balance and tranquility.

The versatility of So-Hum is that it works for recovery after exercise, as well as on the meditation cushion or in everyday stressful situations. Recovery doesn't have to be just after physical exercise. Practice So-Hum at any time when you want to elicit a parasympathetic response. I find myself at the gym after a HIIT session sitting next to kettle bells and the Airdyne, feeling So-Hum vibrate inside of my head. Whether it's after a yoga session, while on my bike, or during moments of stress or anxiety, reciting So-Hum allows me to draw upon the calming and balancing effects of the parasympathetic nervous system.

PRACTICE

So-Hum Mantra for Relaxation

Find a comfortable position, seated or lying down, allowing your spine to lengthen and your body to relax. Gently close your eyes or soften your gaze, directing your attention between your eyebrows. Relax your face, shoulders, and belly.

Set your intention, perhaps thinking: *May all beings everywhere experience deep rest and tranquility.*

Now, bring your awareness to your breath. Take a slow Breath Wave, filling from the bottom and expanding your ribs. As you exhale, release any tension, allowing your body to soften and relax. Place your tongue on your upper palate. Allow your breath to settle into its natural rhythm, observing the gentle rise and fall of each inhalation and exhalation.

As you continue to breathe, quietly or mentally recite the syllable "so" on your inhalation. Allow the vowel to extend for the duration of your inhale, "soooooooooo," feeling its soothing vibration resonating throughout your head and throat.

Allow "so" to encompass the essence of your inhalation, guiding you deep within.

As you exhale, quietly or mentally recite the syllable "hum," feeling its comforting sound, "huuuuuuuummmmmm" reverberating within your skull. Release any tension, letting go of anything that no longer serves you. Allow the "hum" to wash away any burdens, creating space for tranquility and inner peace.

Continue this slow mantra practice of "so" on your inhalation and "hum" on your exhalation. Let the mantra and your breath become a guide in the flow of the ever-changing moment we call now.

Sooooooo on your inhale.

Huuuummm on your exhale.

Continue with the So-Hum practice for as long as you feel fresh and alert.

When you are ready, slowly let go of the mantra recitation. Rest in silent stillness for short while. Feel the mantra continuing to reverberate within you.

Gently open your eyes and carry the tranquility of So-Hum with you.

Whether training, staying fit, or coping with daily stresses, physiological recovery fosters resiliency and strength. Tapping into your innate resilience through breathing and restorative practices optimizes recovery, enabling you to excel amid challenges, both physical and mental. The next chapter will explore the powerful impact of meditation, one of the most parasympathetic-inducing practices available.

KEY INSIGHTS

- Prior to engaging in exercise, take a few minutes to stretch and massage your diaphragm and ribs. This proactive approach readies your respiratory muscles, enhances their flexibility, mitigates the risk of injury, and bolsters blood circulation and oxygen delivery.

- Incorporate the exercise intensity dial (EID) as a guide during your workout to tailor your breathing to match the level of exertion and metabolic demand. Ranging from nasal-only breathing for lower intensities to mouth breathing for heightened intensity, the EID optimizes the efficiency of your breathing mechanics and biochemistry.

- Recognize that recovery is pivotal for adapting and repairing your body following the physical stress of exercise. Adaptations and strength gains occur during the recovery phase, not while exercising. Begin your recovery process promptly by dedicating a few minutes to downregulating, using conscious breathing immediately after your workout.

Chapter 11

BREATHING FOR MEDITATION

I began a formal meditation practice 30 years ago when I first went to the Himalayas. The arc of my three decades of study and practice of meditation has allowed me to learn from teachers in hermitages, monasteries, and caves and along sacred rivers in Tibet, Nepal, India, as well as in the West. Sometimes I meditated with them for a few days, sometimes for months. Sometimes it was basic mindfulness; other times it was esoteric tantric practices. Whether I was with Buddhist nuns and monks in Nepal, yogis along the Bagmati and Ganges rivers, Vipassana teachers in the forests of India, or tummö masters in Tibet, they all began their meditation teachings with similar instruction: place your attention upon the breath.

The principle reason for turning your attention to the breath at the start of a meditation session is because it is meant to not only provide a pattern interrupter to our constant mental chatter but also tune our physical body into a receptive, open, and calm state—what many call a flow state or, as Dr. Andrew Weil states, "the breath is the animated, nonphysical aspect of your being. So that when you look in the direction of breath, when you focus your attention on your breath, you are really looking at your spiritual self."[1]

When we are living in a monastery in the mountains or a meditation hut along a serene river, often it only takes that simple turning of attention toward the breath for a few minutes for calmness to pervade, for us to tap in to the nonphysical aspect of our beings. But for those of us who are taking care of our families, frequently consuming social media and news, moving constantly between work and recreation, focusing our attention on our breath is not sufficient to calm the body and the mind—it's anything but a flow state. Rather, it's a distracted state. And what happens then when we try to meditate when the body and mind are not sufficiently settled is we meet thought loops that constantly distract us. Frustration quickly ensues, and an insight-filled meditation practice remains elusive.

I have taught meditation for more than a dozen years to groups and individuals. One of the most important things that I have found in those thousands of hours of teaching, as well as in my own meditation practice, is how critical it is to prepare your body and mind for meditation. You know from this book that your conscious breathing interventions can be relied on to change your state. You can breathe how you want to feel. Applying this knowledge of how to adjust your state, both physically and mentally before you meditate, is a skillful way to extract all the benefits that await you from this ancient art.

If you already have a meditation practice where you are rarely distracted or don't fall asleep, then you probably don't need to incorporate conscious breathing into your practice. If, on the other hand, like the great majority of us, your meditation practice is punctuated with a thousand distracting thoughts or your energy often sinks into lethargy, then using conscious breathing before and during your meditation will be immensely helpful.

Why concentrate on the breath before a meditation session? If we don't adjust our internal state before meditation, we face the monumental challenge of using the mind to overcome the mind. The thinking mind begins to battle that part of you that seeks a meditative state but is overcome by the thoughts themselves. This begins a battle royale between your thinking mind and your own meditating mind. Does this sound familiar to your meditation practice? Nearly everyone I meet nods in agreement.

I know of no more effective way to prepare ourselves for meditation than utilizing the breath. Yes, there are prayers, mantras, visualizations, and devotional practices that may create a conducive psychophysical environment for meditation. Even so, the breath is the place to start, even if other methods are going to be employed. This is why Jon Kabat-Zinn, the individual most responsible for bringing mindfulness meditation to the mainstream in the West, recommends, first and foremost, getting acquainted with the breath in meditation. By doing so, "we are better able to be aware of our thoughts and feelings . . . and with this awareness comes a feeling of having room to move, of having more options, of being free to choose effective and appropriate responses in stressful situations rather than losing our equilibrium and sense of self as a result of feeling overwhelmed, thrown off balance by our own knee-jerk reactions."[2]

When you want to meditate and have an agitated mind, you know the breathing dials from Chapter 3 to turn down to regulate your nervous system. If you are tired and want to meditate, you know how to upregulate so you don't nod off. And even during your meditation session, should you need to insert a breathing intervention to change your state, you have that at the ready. Your breathing tool kit sets you up for the promise of meditation—insights, clarity, focus, relaxed spaciousness, and a journey to discover the nature of consciousness. You have the power.

Breathing Before Meditation

Using the AIR approach, when you set aside time to meditate, I advise you first to check how you feel. This is not complicated, but it is necessary to become aware of how you feel in body and mind, right here, right now, and adjust appropriately before you meditate.

It might be helpful to give an example of what happens when you don't first become aware of your state and just dive into a breathing intervention. Before the pandemic, I regularly practiced a very energizing form of breathing in the morning before meditation. I turned my breathing dials way up for about 20 minutes, cycling through a few rounds of a vigorous, quick pace at nearly maximum volume, and I'd hold my breath for long durations after both exhaling and inhaling—hallmarks of an upregulating breathing practice. And it worked as expected. I'd finish feeling supercharged, completely awake and focused for a meditation session, which I did even before pulling a shot from my beloved espresso machine.

Then the pandemic came, and like others, I experienced stress unlike any before, waking up in the middle of the night worried about my friends and family. Throughout the day, I was stressed about the air all around me! In the evening, my wife and I discussed people we knew who were sick or dying.

When I got up in the morning during this period for my breathing and meditation, I didn't check in with my state, how I was feeling. This was a mistake. I did what I'd been doing for a few years—using the breath to turn up my sympathetic nervous system for laser clarity and energy, to power through the day. The difference was that my nervous system was already stressed in an excessively aroused state, approaching a fight-or-flight response, and the upregulating breathing for 20 minutes only intensified it, tipping me over the edge. My meditation sessions after the breathing were marked by agitation, and I found myself uncharacteristically nervous throughout the day, including having heart palpitations. This is an example of an unskillful way to use breathing practices.

So, before your meditation begins, check in with yourself: Do you need to calm your stormy and agitated mind? Do you need more energy to concentrate? Are you feeling well balanced and want to open yourself to your inner landscape? Once you are aware of your inner state, you initiate a breathing intervention for a few minutes—enough to shift your internal state. As you know, you'll be adjusting your biochemistry, your blood gases, and the delivery of energy that prepares your body and mind for meditation. This may be turning up the sympathetic nervous system more than the parasympathetic, or vice versa, or balancing the two with just enough focus and concentration not to be distracted but enough relaxation to recline your mind. You are in charge. Breathe how you want to meditate!

I'm going to offer two suggested breathing practices that have long been used as a preliminary to meditation in the Buddhist and yogic traditions. Depending on your state, use one of these two practices before meditation: either Alternate Nostril Breathing for balancing and relaxation or Skull Shining Breathing to upregulate the nervous system.

Before we learn these two breathing practices, I want to address one of the most common questions I receive about meditation because it is relevant to not only formal meditation and breathing practice, but life in general: *What am I supposed to do with all these thoughts?*

What to Do with All These Thoughts?

An essential part of any meditation practice is to notice what is moving across the landscape of our minds, like thoughts, emotions, and perception in general. Sometimes a thought arises and passes, and we don't think about it, like a bird whose flight path leaves no trace in the sky. Other times, thoughts arise in our mind, and we start to think about them. Sometimes we notice right away when we start thinking; other times we might not even realize how long we've been away on a thought loop. In meditation, an important element is noticing when we've moved away from what we are concentrating on, such as the breath.

What do we do when we notice we are distracted? What do we do when we catch ourselves thinking? We simply release the thinking, relax, and return to the breath.

Release, relax, and return to the practice—it seems so simple. Yet again and again we run up against our own entrenched habit of chasing our thoughts. So, each time we notice, we have to do it again: release, relax, and return to the practice. Like any mental skill, it takes practice.

When we notice we are distracted, there's no need to think about why we were thinking, because this is, of course, another layer of thinking, which is not our intention at this time. We don't have to do anything except release the thinking, relax, and return.

The consequence of returning our attention to our meditation is that worries, fears, and stress are released.

Each time we notice our distractions, we are given an opportunity to relax.

There is a subtle but important point that I want to highlight. In meditation, we're not trying to block thoughts. The notion of "emptying the mind" or "thought-free awareness" is a fallacy. Thoughts will continue to arise as long as we are alive. But in meditation, we are releasing ourselves from thinking about those thoughts. If we try to block and suppress thoughts, or have some idea that meditation should somehow dissolve thoughts altogether, we'll become frustrated very quickly. So, instead, when thoughts or emotions arise, we release the thinking about them.

When we release and relax, a thought may seem to linger, even though we aren't thinking about it. It is not unlike when a child lets go of a helium-filled balloon—it hovers for a time but gradually drifts away. Thoughts are the same. If thoughts seem to linger for longer than we like, a dose of patience and kindness toward ourselves is helpful.

Release, relax, and return to your breath with joy.

Alternate Nostril Breathing to Prepare for Meditation

The breathing practice below is known as Alternate Nostril Breathing. This is a centuries-old pranayama practice to bring clarity in mind and balance the flow of energy in the body in preparation for meditation. The balance comes from gently turning up both wings of your autonomic nervous system, just enough sympathetic and parasympathetic nervous systems activation.[3,¶¶¶] This is accomplished in the practice by the release of the right amount of noradrenaline,

---

¶¶¶   Alternate Nostril Breathing is known as *Nadi Shodhana* in Sanskrit. *Nadi* means "energy channel," and *Shodhana* means "to purify." Alternate Nostril Breathing is generally safe and beneficial for most people, including children and the elderly. If you have had recent nasal surgery or have an active nostril infection, please consult your doctor.

a hormone triggering a sympathetic nervous system response. Researchers at the Trinity College Institute of Neuroscience and the Global Brain Health Institute in Dublin, Ireland, found that slow, controlled, deep breathing—like we are going to do with Alternate Nostril Breathing—helps the brain find the noradrenaline "sweet spot," increasing attention and getting us laser focused. A similar degree of noradrenaline is released when we are engaged with deep curiosity or passion, all of which promotes the growth of neural connections in the brain.[4] This research showed that performing Alternate Nostril Breathing after learning a motor skill improves both immediate and long-term retention of that skill.

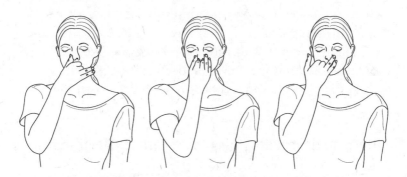

ALTERNATE NOSTRIL BREATHING

The practice involves alternating the breath between either nostril, using your ring finger and thumb to gently close one nostril at a time while inhaling or exhaling through the other.

PRACTICE

Alternate Nostril Breathing

- Find a comfortable seated position on the floor or in a chair. Lean back if you wish but keep your back upright and relaxed. Place your tongue on your upper palate and relax your face.

- Set your intention: *May my breathing practice today bring me clarity, focus, and relaxation so that I spread positivity in my family and community.*

- Turn your attention to how you feel at this time. Just notice.

- Begin your Alternate Nostril Breathing. With your right hand, bring your index finger and middle finger to rest between your eyebrows. Gently close your right nostril with your right thumb and slowly inhale through your left nostril. Feel the breath flowing in smoothly and steadily.

- After the inhale, pause for a moment, release your thumb, close your left nostril with your ring finger, and exhale slowly and completely through your right nostril. Feel the breath leaving your body with a sense of release and relaxation.

- Keeping your left nostril closed, inhale through your right nostril. Experience the breath entering your body, bringing in fresh energy and clarity. Pause for a moment.

- After the inhale, close your right nostril with your thumb while releasing your ring finger from your left nostril, and exhale through your left nostril. Feel the breath flowing out effortlessly, carrying away any tension or stress.

- This completes one round of Alternate Nostril Breathing. Continue the practice for 10 to 15 more rounds.

- As you continue the practice, maintain a smooth, steady breath. Focus your attention on the sensation of the breath as it enters and leaves your body. Feel the calming and balancing effects as you synchronize your breath.

- Gradually, with each round, try to extend the duration of the breath, making the inhales and exhales longer and smoother. Take your time and listen to your body's natural rhythm.

- Practice for 10 minutes, or as long as feels comfortable for you.

- When you're ready to conclude, release your fingers from your forehead. Rest for a few moments and feel the effects of the practice.

Adjust the practice of Alternate Nostril Breathing in the following ways to increase your energy or for relaxation.

To stimulate more energy:

- Slightly increase the pace and volume of your inhale.

- Hold your breath after every inhale for a 5 count.

To bring about more calm:

- Extend the exhale for twice as long as the inhale.

- Hold your breath after every exhale for a 5 count.

Skull Shining Breathing

Skull Shining Breathing supercharges your entire system.**** The practice is a vigorous, energetic technique that tones the abdominal wall and activates the respiratory musculature. In the practice, we use a forceful, rhythmic bellow-pumping on the exhalation, which stirs dormant and sluggish energy, especially in the pelvic bowl, and moves it upward within the body.

In our normal breathing, the inhalation is more active and the exhalation is passive. Skull Shining Breathing reverses this order. We make the exhalation active by forcefully driving the abdominal wall toward the spine. This action is performed by a sudden, forceful strike—contracting the abdominal muscles to drive the air out.

After you have expelled the air, the inhalation happens passively because of the vacuum in the lung. This reflexive inhalation is three to four times as long as the active exhalation—allow the inhalation to happen on its own. The ratio of this longer, passive inhalation with the forceful exhalation is the hallmark of Skull Shining Breathing.

When learning the practice, find control with a very slow pace and a definitive strike of the exhalation. Speeding up too quickly leads to shallow, superficial strikes, which have little effect. It is important to do the exercise slowly and methodically.

The most common mistake in Skull Shining Breathing is to make the inhalation active or to not allow the passive inhale to complete itself. Make the striking exhalation and the passive inhalation completely separate events. Try to relax the belly after each vigorous abdominal strike. One might tire quickly, so it is important to maintain the quality of strikes.

**** The Sanskrit name for this practice is *kapalabhati pranayama*, and some breathing schools in the West have renamed it as Breath of Fire because of the energy it generates.

During the practice, focus your attention halfway between the navel and pubic bone. If it feels comfortable, you might lightly pull up on your pelvic floor. The seated posture should be very steady, so be sure that your hips, thighs, and knees are supported by cushions—they should not be bouncing during the practice. Refrain from lifting the shoulders when passively inhaling and also keep the head steady with the face relaxed.

PRACTICE

Skull Shining Breathing

- Sit comfortably and stable, making sure your hips and knees are supported under a cushion.

- Relax the face and shoulders, and place the tongue on the upper palate.

- Set your intention, perhaps thinking: *May I energize my body and mind so that I may be fully present and loving with my family and community.*

- Turn your attention to how you feel at this time. Just notice.

- Begin Skull Shining Breathing. Inhale normally.

- Exhale with a sharp strike of your belly toward your spine.

- Allow a passive inhale to return.

- Strike your exhale.

- Allow a passive inhale.

- Make the striking exhale and passive inhale separate events.

- Continue for 20 to 30 strikes, allowing the passive inhale to return each time and relaxing your face and shoulders. No need to rush.

- After 20 to 30 Skull Shining strikes, inhale fully and hold for a 5 to 10 count, your attention resting in your heart.

- Relax the face, jaw, and shoulders.

- Slowly exhale through the nose.

Repeat for 3 to 5 rounds.

- After your last round, let go and rest in silent stillness. Feel the effects of the practice.

8 Tips for Establishing a Daily Breath and Meditation Practice

I have found enormous benefits from meditating daily for the last 30 years. It's not easy establishing a daily routine of meditation, conscious breathing, yoga, or any other activity where we traverse our internal landscape. It's a challenge to be consistent. Here are my 8 tips for establishing a daily breathing and meditation practice.

1. **Remind yourself of your motivation.**

    Write in your journal or on a piece of paper your motivation for your conscious breathing and meditation practice. Use this as a reminder before each session. Perhaps write a new motivation from time to time.

2. Do short sessions, many times.

Keep your sessions on the shorter side, especially at the beginning. Breathe and meditate daily for 5 to 15 minutes. The point is to practice with relaxed alertness and to change your state. It is more beneficial to have a short session that brings you joy and a feeling of being alive than it is to meditate sleepily for 45 minutes. Try to conclude your session when you are still fresh and wouldn't mind continuing. Slowly increase the length and frequency of formal sessions but not past the point of freshness. As for how to keep track of how long you meditate or practice conscious breathing, I recommend having a clock in the room that is not on your smartphone (leave your phone outside your meditation space). Sand timers work great.

3. Keep your practice close to your heart.

My first Tibetan Buddhist meditation teacher told me, "Don't tell anyone you meditate." I didn't understand immediately what he meant, but today I do. In the beginning, sometimes our enthusiasm takes over, and we talk a lot about practice but meditate or employ breathing interventions very little. Consider redirecting that enthusiastic energy inward to fuel your practice. That said, it's good to let your partner or close friends know what you're doing so they lend support as you establish a regular practice. And finding a community of breathers or meditators for regular practice together is very powerful.

4. **Establish a routine.**

We form habits very quickly—both positive and negative. We can use this tendency to our advantage in our daily breath and meditation practice by establishing a routine. Associate your new practice with something you enjoy. Perhaps you breathe and meditate immediately after your coffee or tea is made. Or right after your yoga practice—each time. One of my friends waits in her church pew at the end of the service to breathe and meditate. Perhaps your days are so full that you need to schedule your formal session in your daily planner—if so, schedule it. Initially it will take some effort and discipline, but soon your interest increases with the felt benefit, and you'll establish the habit. Strive on, with ease, because it is like the Buddha said in the Fundamentals of the Path, "A disciplined mind brings happiness."

5. **Commit.**

Make a commitment to a formal breath and meditation session each day for a certain period. You can write it down in your journal, for example: "I will breathe and meditate for 10 minutes every day for the next month." Go easy on yourself, though—remember, short sessions, many times. It is better to meditate for 5 to 10 minutes every day for a month than for one hour on a random weekend. One of my teachers says that establishing a daily meditation practice "is like brushing your teeth—we do it a few times each day, rather than waiting until Sunday and brushing for an hour. If you do that, it will be painful, not very useful, and you'll probably see some blood! Every day you brush—every day you meditate."

6. **Practice when you practice.**

When you sit down to breathe and meditate in a formal session, just do that. There's no need to check your e-mail on your smartphone one last time. Or to stretch your body extensively. When it's time to practice, just practice. Body still. Speech silent. Mind spacious and alert. No need to waste time arranging this and that and taking the long road to the zafu.

7. **Keep a book of insights.**

Note down in your journal what you practiced and any insights that arose during your session. Every so often, reread your insights as a reminder to yourself.

8. **Rejoice!**

At the conclusion of your daily breath and meditation practice, before jumping off your cushion and rushing into your day, savor the moment. In this solitary time, rejoice and offer gratitude for the fortunate circumstances that allow you to cultivate a path of insight and meditation. Remember that you are blessed to have this opportunity. Rejoicing in our own and others' good fortune is a way of energizing our practice. Even after meditation or breath sessions that we have found challenging or boring, we can rejoice that we've made a sustained effort to cultivate clarity of mind and softness of heart.

Breathing into Nonduality

The practice I'd like to share with you now is called Spacious Outbreath. This is a fusion of meditation and breathing practices, where we shift our focus from a specific object of concentration, such as the coarse breath or a sensation, to a more expansive awareness. We rest our attention in the spacious gap after the exhalation, and this allows for deep relaxation while remaining attentive. Your breath is your trusted guide.

As we immerse ourselves in the Spacious Outbreath, we have the potential to glimpse a profound state of concept-free awareness. This practice is not about spacing out; rather, it is an invitation to abide in a heightened state of awareness without fixating on anything in particular. We allow our breath to guide us on this journey into what some call a nondual state, beyond thoughts and thinking.

During Spacious Outbreath practice, we may experience a sense of boundlessness, free of limits. In the openness, we might also notice how thinking restricts our boundless awareness, tightening us. Recognizing this, we understand how our thoughts bind us and impede our ability to see reality as it is without distortion or preconceived notions. By cultivating this panoramic awareness, we develop a useful detachment from situations and emotions that typically elicit negative reactions in us.

Detachment should not be mistaken for indifference or disconnection. On the contrary, it enables us to see our ever-changing inner landscape and the external world with clarity, empowering us to act with compassion for ourselves and others.

The Spacious Outbreath practice has a profound calming effect on both the body and mind, sometimes even inducing drowsiness. While we strive to strike a balance between attentiveness and relaxation, drowsiness is a common obstacle. To counter this, I offer some suggestions: straighten your spine, adjust your physical posture, open your underarms to cool down, allow fresh air into the room, try meditating with your eyes open, ensure you have had enough sleep, and if needed, enjoy a cup of tea or coffee before your practice.

PRACTICE

Spacious Outbreath

Find a comfortable seated position on the floor or in a chair, or lie down if you're experiencing any bodily discomfort. Create a stable foundation by grounding yourself. Lengthen your spine and gently tuck your chin. If your eyes are open, cast your gaze downward or softly close them. Completely relax the muscles in your face and shoulders, allowing your belly to be loose and free from tension.

Set your intention, perhaps with: *May this meditation cultivate an open heart and a clear mind, enabling me to engage with my family and community with love.*

Having settled in comfortable stillness, bring your awareness into your body. Feel its stability and downward pull of gravity. For a few moments, let your attention hover within and around your body, noticing the most prominent sensations. Deepen your relaxation.

Now, gently redirect your attention to your breath. Identify where you perceive your breath most distinctly—whether it's around your nostrils, in your chest, or within your belly. Rest your attention there. Observe the rising inhalation and the descending exhalation. Notice the texture and length of your breath, allowing it to flow naturally while maintaining a witnessing mode of attention.

As you continue to relax your body and observe your breath, shift your focus to the end of your exhalation. Watch the breath go out and notice the gap. No need to hold your breath or alter its flow; simply observe the brief pause, the space, as the exhale dissolves into space.

Rest within the expansive outbreath, and as you inhale, follow the breath inward.

Again, as your awareness rides the breath outward, there's no need to exert any effort. Abide in the spaciousness at the end of the outbreath, remaining alert and open.

You may become aware of sounds, thoughts, or external occurrences. That's no problem. Your body remains still, breath natural, and mind relaxed yet attentive. Continue to explore the Spacious Outbreath, allowing your breath to flow naturally like the ebb and flow of a vast ocean.

When thoughts arise or distractions occur, gently bring your attention back to your breath. Observe it a few times, in and out, and then, on an outbreath, once again let go into the spacious gap at the end of the breath. Practice in this manner for the next 10 to 15 minutes.

During this time, avoid attempting to block or suppress anything. Allow the world around you to arise and pass, and thoughts to come and go, while remaining focused on your breath and repeatedly resting in the expansive gap at the end of each outbreath.

> To conclude your practice, release any mental effort of concentrating on the breath. Completely relax in silent stillness for a few minutes.

Expanding the Effortless Pause

After practicing breathing exercises like Alternate Nostril Breathing, Spacious Outbreath, or the Letting Go AH Practice in the next chapter, you may notice a spontaneous but temporary suspension of breathing. This is not the unconscious breath holding brought on by stress that we discussed earlier. Instead, there is neither inhalation nor exhalation, but there is also no effort involved in holding the breath, sometimes for a few moments or even minutes. The breath suspends itself.

From the yogic perspective, this effortless pause in breathing, known in the ancient texts as *kevala kumbhaka*, or pure retention, is cherished because of the sensation of being beyond linear time and the opportunity it offers for spiritual realizations.[5] Maybe you have felt this effortless breath suspension, but no one ever named the experience. One of my pranayama teachers in India described *kevala kumbhaka* as "the fourth time" because there is a sense of hovering not in the past, future, or even present but only the expanding sensation of boundless awareness. This treasured opportunity, according to the sage Ramana Maharshi, is where release from mental and physical suffering occurs, if only momentarily.[6]

Whenever this graceful and unforced gap emerges, "you have arrived at the pinnacle, so there is no need to do anything at all," my teacher instructed. It might happen after deep relaxation, during a breathing intervention, while meditating, or sometimes upon concluding chanting or humming for an extended period—the breath seems to be so slight that there is no movement. When this happens, let your awareness dissolve into limitless space, as though a clay pot has broken into pieces and the space within merges with the outer expanse. This natural suspension of the breath may feel like entering a portal to another dimension. Master Eckhart, the 13th-century German philosopher, tries to put the experience to words, writing, "there is a place inside of you that neither time, nor space, nor no created thing can ever touch."

This effortless suspension also happens during moments of awe or after sexual intercourse, which is in part why the French call the post-orgasm glide *la petite mort*, a little death. Another such instance is immediately after a sneeze. As the sneeze subsides, direct your awareness to the space that follows, delving into the momentary pause, exploring the openness and clarity that emerges. Similarly, when you find yourself on the verge of falling asleep or waking up, embrace that delicate in-between state—often there will be no movement of breath. Hover on the edge of consciousness, fully present in the realm of transition. Here, you connect with the boundless potentiality that resides within this liminal space.

When you find yourself dropping into this nondual state, free and spontaneous breath suspension, relax and let go completely for however long it lasts. It's an invitation into pure being. As Rainer Maria Rilke wrote in *Letters to a Young Poet*, "Go into yourself and see how deep the place is from which your life flows."

The connection between this place from which life flows, your breath, and death is where we are going in the next chapters.

KEY INSIGHTS

- Set yourself up to fulfill the promise of meditation by preparing your body and mind with conscious breathing before you meditate. If you need to down-regulate, use Alternate Nostril Breathing; if you need energy to focus, use Skull Shining Breathing.

- When you notice you're distracted while meditating, release the thinking, relax the body, and return to the breath. Each time. Release, relax, and return to the breath.

- If you find your breath spontaneously suspends itself, where there is no inhalation or exhalation or effort to hold your breath, allow your awareness to merge with the expanse of space.

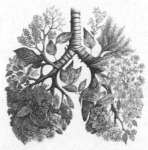

Part III

BREATHE HOW YOU WANT TO DIE

Chapter 12

LETTING GO WITH
THE BREATH

You have spent the better part of this book delving into ways to adjust your breathing so that you breathe how you want to feel. You have learned different breathing techniques and practices so your life flourishes, so that you are fully present with your loved ones. You have a robust breathing tool kit now to respond with skill and agility to the ever-changing circumstances of your life.

Sometimes you need to dial up your energy; other times you need to downregulate in response to an acute stressor. As your ability grows to sense the interiority of your emotional landscape and feeling tone, you're able to change your state on demand within a few cycles of breathing. You know how to self-regulate your nervous system throughout the day with your breathing so that restorative sleep happens at night. Consistently breathing optimally day-to-day, during exercise and meditation, is the foundation for your health and well-being. You know how to breathe how you want to live.

While being able to breathe how you want to feel has been the focus of this book, the fact remains that one day, you, like everyone else, will breathe your last breath. Bridging to the topic of death might seem shocking after all that we've previously covered. But there is nothing more real than death. And when death is imminent, there are no adjustments or breathing interventions that prevent its eventuality. When the dying process begins, there will only be you, your awareness, and what remains after your breath stops. To breathe how we want to feel ultimately means we breathe how we want to die.

In coming chapters, we are going to prepare for dying by contemplating mortality and meditating on our own death. Thinking about mortality does not have to be depressing, nor does it lower your vibration or stoke for life. Still, it's never easy for any of us to contemplate death. But connecting with the truth about the fragility and impermanent nature of existence helps us prioritize. Thinking about death spurs us to seize each day with joy and gratitude so that we die peacefully with no regrets. As the visionary cofounder of the Zen Hospice Project, Frank Ostaseski, says in *The Five Invitations: Discovering What Death Can Teach Us About Living Fully*, "death is not waiting for us at the end of a long road. Death is always with us, in the marrow of every passing moment. She is the secret teacher hiding in plain sight. She helps us to discover what matters most. And the good news is we don't have to wait until the end of our lives to realize the wisdom that death has to offer."[1]

Just consider for a moment, how will you be when you breathe your last breath?

Imagine for a few moments, right now, how it will feel when you exhale, and the breath does not return.

What emotions move through you when you consider your breath ceasing forever?

How does your body feel when you think about your impending death?

What happens to your breathing at this moment while contemplating your mortality?

You may have never considered these questions. The first time I was asked these kinds of questions, fear immediately gripped me. Seven out of ten of us feel uncomfortable when considering our own death.[2] But sages and wisdom keepers across cultures and spiritual traditions converge on the singular point that to think frequently about your mortality—while you are healthy—is extremely beneficial to finding what is most meaningful in life. A Greek proverb tells us, "Death is not the greatest loss in life. The greatest loss is what dies inside us while we live."

Death is an undeniable presence woven into the fabric of our existence, whether we consciously think about it or not. It is in the background of our lives, making its presence more apparent when a loved one dies, when obituaries appear in the church newsletters, or reports of natural disasters catch our attention during a news cycle. Death influences unconscious choices we make throughout the day: what we eat, why we exercise, and how we plan our financial future. This ever-present yet concealed reality of death compels us to take our child's hand as we cross the street or buckle a life preserver before paddling in a canoe. It's the motivation behind putting a bicycle helmet on, flipping the blinker on before turning onto the highway, and looking both ways before crossing a street. Even though dying may not be in the forefront of my thinking, it's why I leash myself to my surfboard when I paddle out into the ocean.

Thinking about death actively, to explore our emotional interiority through the lens of mortality, is not something that most of us are used to doing. But that's where we are headed in these next chapters. Modern society doesn't encourage it but rather works hard to obscure it, redirecting our attention to the shiny and suggesting deep meaning is to be found in the new. From the technological devices we use to the clothing we wear, from the toys and entertainment for the young and old, to even our own skin, society pushes our attention toward the novel and youthful rather than finding meaning in the worn and aged.

~≈

When I first moved to Kathmandu in my early 20s, I lived close to the Bagmati River, considered a sacred waterway of the Himalayas. The river was where locals brought their deceased to be cremated along the banks near Pashupatinath Temple. Every day I saw processions of a dozen or so people carrying shrouded corpses to the river. At the water's edge, there were wood pyres upon which the bodies were laid. While prayers were recited, the body was anointed with blessed oil and orange marigold flowers were scattered. Then the flame was lit. After a few hours, ashes were swept into the water.

I was studying with a Buddhist nun who encouraged me to use the experience of seeing the dead bodies as a reminder of my own mortality and realize the truth of impermanence.†††† She had given me a text where the Buddha taught, "Of all footprints, the elephant's is supreme. Of all meditations, remembering death and impermanence is supreme." Another book I studied encouraged us to become intimate with death now, while the body and mind are sound. "Warned of a hurricane, we don't

---

†††† The Buddhist meditation practice on death is called *maranassati*. While mentioned frequently in scriptures, the most prominent scripture is the *Maranassati Sutta*. A commentary offered on the practice can be found in the *Visuddhimagga (Path of Purification)* by Buddhaghosa.

wait until the storm pounds the shore before we start to prepare. Similarly, knowing death is looming offshore, we shouldn't wait until it overpowers us before developing the meditative skills necessary to achieve the great potential of the mind at the moment of death."[3]

After a few months in the home where I was living with a family in Kathmandu, the matriarch of the household died. I was invited into her bedroom where she lay. While I had been to funerals in America, it was the first time in my life I'd seen a dead body. Like many Americans, unless we work in emergency services, the military, hospitals, hospices, morgues, or graveyards, there is little chance to meet death face-to-face in everyday life.

I joined a dozen other family members in the room. A local Tibetan Buddhist monk arrived and quietly prayed next to the grandmother, whom they had propped up, as if she were sitting in meditation. Her eyes were sunken and cheeks more prominent than the day before. Though her breath may have stopped, Tibetan Buddhists believe that the consciousness is still present within the body for a time. In this liminal period where the mind is no longer tied to experience by the physical senses, spiritual realization more readily unfolds.

On the first day, the monk occasionally whispered in the ear of the elderly woman, "You are dying. You lived well. Let go of whatever arises in your mind. Release and let go." The monk told the family to pray silently, but if they needed to express grief and cry aloud, they should move into another room so as not to create distress for the dying grandmother, who was in the process of letting go of her body. As the monk sat next to the body for three days, life continued in the house, with folks cooking, others tending to the babies, and others praying. On the fourth day, the monk pulled on a tuft of hair on the crown of the grandmother's head. Afterward he said the consciousness had exited from the body. The dying process was finished. The family washed the body with saffron water and carried it down to the river to be cremated. It was the first time I watched the body of someone I had known burn. I meditated on the inevitability of my own body being reduced to dust.

During my first year of living in Nepal, I meditated daily on death awareness that the nun taught me. Sometimes I meditated along the riverbank with smoke in the distance; other times it was in my room. The form that the practice took was twofold: first, the Nine Contemplations on Death, and secondly, I prepared for my own death with a Death Rehearsal Meditation. We will explore both of these practices in the pages to come.

The Great Mystery

In all cultures, death has been a *mysterium tremendum,* an awe-inspiring mystery. It is likely that religions arose in part to help people cope with the existential anxiety. What happens after death remains pure speculation, whether from a scientific or religious perspective, but the speculation may help mediate death anxiety. We know death is far more than a mere medical event. The profundity of what occurs during the dying process transcends any medical, philosophical, or religious model. The dying process shakes loose all layers of our self-definition. We feel our persona cultivated throughout our life dissolving from within. This persona and associated identities gracefully surrender or are stripped away by sickness and death.

It may seem like a paradox that the only way to fully embrace life is to courageously embrace the unknowable reality of our death. It is in recognizing how ephemeral our very existence is that we can know its preciousness.

For those with a purely secular, materialist view of the world, death negates and terminates being; our existence and consciousness abruptly cease at the moment of death followed by absolute and eternal nothingness. This reductionist belief holds that there is no movement of soul, spirit, energy, or consciousness—whatever you may call what is at the basis of who you are beyond death.

Mainstream medical care around the world is implicitly influenced by this materialist attitude, which partially explains why doctors try to heroically stave off or postpone death for as long as possible. This may contribute to why only half of Americans over age 65 have ever considered how they want to die.[4] It could be argued that this perennial battle against death is modern medicine's primary *raison d'être*. I'm not suggesting that we should not avail ourselves to the extraordinary healing potential and pain mitigation that Western medicine provides. I am extremely thankful for the life-extending treatments both my mother and father received upon their cancer diagnosis.

Still, we cannot deny that society strives desperately to control, suppress, and defeat death at all costs, even at the price of the dying patient's dignity. "By focusing on fixes, we ignore finitude," which is a grave mistake, according to Dr. L.S. Dugale, director of the Center for Clinical Medical Ethics at Columbia University and author of *The Lost Art of Dying: Reviving Forgotten Wisdom*. Dr. Dugale argues that if we carry with us a salient sense of finitude, embrace our fears about death, accept how our bodies age, develop meaningful rituals, and incorporate our communities in end-of-life care, we rediscover what it means to both live and die well.

"The threat of our finitude should drive us toward those we love . . . to die well requires that we live well, and we live best in the company of communities that help us make sense of our finitude and find beauty in decay."[5] But if we ignore the reality of the finitude, death anxiety is likely to manifest.

Acknowledging Death Anxiety

If we choose to contemplate death, as we will do in this chapter, it is not surprising that a certain level of resistance, even anxiety, might arise. Especially when we move beyond the intellectual notion of our death and feel it deeply within our being. You may have felt a stir of unease already, even fear, reading this chapter. We call this death anxiety.

Death anxiety is a very real emotion, and nobody should feel shame if it arises. Death anxiety is the fear of your own death or the suffering that may accompany dying. It might emerge when we are navigating the challenges of surviving, growing, and raising a family and we feel the world is constantly presenting existential threats. Life, beyond its daily stresses, possesses fragility and a tenuousness. When we feel this inherent precariousness, not only in our own life but also in the lives of our family and friends, death anxiety may arise.

What are we to do with this anxiety?

Death anxiety is feedback from within. And this feedback is energy for inquiry. This is not about overcoming the fear of death but rather being very present with discomfort and how that informs who we are and how we show up in the world.

This might be an opportune time to remember AIR—awareness, intervention, regulation. When you feel fear or angst with the thought of death, that emotion is a signal or movement within your awareness, the first step in AIR. Before actively contemplating death, you have tools in your breathing tool kit to initiate a breathing intervention to calm your racing heart, fretful mind, or other manifestation of death anxiety. And then as you continue to think about mortality, you regulate your nervous system if needed. The breath is your very reliable ally. As you move forward in these pages, take your time and use your breath to keep you centered and calm. And if you feel overwhelmed, you might put this book down for some time, talk to a loved one about your feelings, journal, or be outside in nature with your breath.

Thinking about death is not about stirring a sense of dread. Rather, embracing the truth of mortality diminishes anxiety about our own and our loved one's death. And this helps us be present with others during their dying process and friends and family who are grieving. Contemplating death helps reduce the suffering of attachment and emotional reactivity to change in general, increases a sense of gratitude for daily existence, and cultivates a greater compassion for oneself and other people.

That said, meditating on death is not for everyone. For those suffering from trauma, severe depression, or psychological instability, please consult a healthcare or mental health professional before proceeding.

Practicing Memento Mori

Numerous cultures around the world have embraced formal contemplations on death as an antidote to death anxiety. From Socrates to the Buddha to the Old Testament, there is an urging to recognize the preciousness of life and its inherent brevity. One such tradition rooted in Greco-Roman antiquity is encapsulated in the Latin phrase *memento mori*—"remember, you will die." Stoics embraced memento mori and encouraged living each day as if it were your last. Memento mori is a mental training that hits bone deep. It changes the way we see the world. And when we change the way we see the world, the world itself changes.

Incorporating memento mori into our daily lives enhances our resilience. By acknowledging the certainty of death, we listen to our fears and learn to embrace uncertainty. It shifts our perspective from dwelling on future worries to fully embracing the present. Memento mori teaches us to let go of attachments, including material possessions and societal expectations, allowing us to live unbound and authentically. We gain a renewed sense of urgency to pursue our passions, take risks, and stop procrastinating, knowing that every moment is a precious gift. We see that death reveals to us what is most dear. Thinking of death, we love more.

An active training of memento mori can take the shape of punctuating our day with a mental recitation of the phrase, "remember, I will die," and the potency of its meaning. Alua Arthur, death doula and author of *Briefly Perfectly Human: Making an Authentic Life by Getting Real about the End*, suggests looking deeply into your own eyes in the mirror while reciting the phrase and observing compassionately what emotions arise. In this sense, memento mori is used like a mantra. Mantras are phrases that tether our mind to a beneficial emotion or thought like love or compassion.

PRACTICE

Memento Mori Mantra

- Synchronize your breath with the mantra: *Memento mori—remember, I will die.*

- Anywhere you find yourself during the day or evening, turn your attention to your breath.

- A single breath is a microcosm of life, emerging and then dissolving into infinity.

- Inhaling, you silently recite, "Remember."

- Notice the pause.

- Exhaling, letting go, you silently recite, "I will die."

- The disappearing exhale offers you a direct and visceral experience of impermanence.

- Embrace and listen to the emotions that well from within as you synchronize the mantra with your breath.

Each time you recall memento mori or follow your exhale to its natural conclusion, you let go of the things that do not serve you, prioritize what does matter, and live in a way that aligns with your values and beliefs. In other words, memento mori is not all about preparing for death. Rather, it is living with an awareness of death which spurs us to embrace life. Life and death are not two separate occurrences but part of a greater wholeness of who we are.

Shortly after the famous psychologist Abraham Maslow almost died from a heart attack, he wrote in a letter, "The confrontation with death—and the reprieve from it—makes everything look so precious, so sacred, so beautiful that I feel more strongly than ever the impulse to love it, to embrace it, and to let myself be overwhelmed by it. Death, and its ever-present possibility, makes love, passionate love, more possible."[6]

When we keep death close at hand, we tend to hold less tightly to our own opinions, take ourselves less seriously, and let go with greater ease so that we connect with others. A natural prioritization of what is meaningful in our life arises from our memento mori training. This prioritization may manifest in your spiritual practice, or you may increase attentive time with those who are near and dear, or perhaps you'll immerse yourself more in nature, or simply love and appreciate the unfolding of your life. As W. Somerset Maugham wrote in *The Razor's Edge*, "Nothing in the world is permanent, and we're foolish when we ask anything to last, but surely we're still more foolish not to take delight in it while we have it."

Letting Go AH Practice

A powerful daily breathing practice that includes an awareness of your own mortality is the Letting Go AH Practice. This practice, building upon the previous chapter's Spacious Outbreath Practice, mingles your breath awareness, in particular your exhalation, with space.

In the Letting Go AH Practice, you begin by feeling the space within your body and head, then you notice the feeling of space around your body and in the room. Continuing outward, you move your attention to the space extending in all directions around you, to the far reaches of the cosmos. After recognizing and expanding your awareness into the space (not becoming spaced out), within and around you, the AH method is employed. On an exhale, softly aspirate the sound *AHHHHH*. You don't say "ah" but rather sigh the sound so that it is lightly audible, loud enough that someone next to you can hear.

At the end of the sound *ah*, you remain motionless (no need to look here and there or even swallow), with nothing to do but expand into the felt spaciousness. Breathing suspended, feel your awareness merging with space outside of you, like water being poured into water. This is a profound practice of not doing, of opening and allowing, of resting in spacious awareness.

As you remain and expand into space, if there is the return of breath with an inhale, that is fine. Let the breath return. If there is an effortless suspension in breathing for some time, that is fine too. Then, after a few minutes of resting in breath awareness, once again employ the AH method. This isn't a recitation practice; there is no set timing. If you notice especially strong thoughts or emotions, or if you catch yourselves in repeated thought loops, that is an appropriate time to use the AH method to dissolve the thought or emotion. And then rest open, spacious, without strain or effort.

PRACTICE

Letting Go AH

- Find a comfortable position, seated or lying down.

- Set your intention: *May my Letting Go AH Practice release any tension or stress so that I may more effectively serve my family and community.*

- Practice breath awareness. Place your attention on the movement of your inhalation and exhalation for a minute.

- Let go of focusing on your breath and notice the feeling of the space inside your head. Your brain occupies the space, but notice the space itself.

- Notice the space inside your torso. Again, there are organs present, but feel the space.

- Feel the space inside your stomach.

- Feel the space inside your legs.

- Move your awareness of space outside your body, about a handspan beyond your head and body in all directions. Feel the space.

- Extend your awareness and feel the space up to the ceiling and to the walls around you.

- Extend your awareness further to the sky up to the clouds, and a few miles in all directions, including below you into the earth. The space has objects temporarily in it but feel the space.

- And finally, feel the space in all directions well beyond the Earth's atmosphere. Feel the expanse of space.

- You will now employ the AH method.

- On an exhale, aspirate *AHHHHH*. Merge your awareness with silence and space.

- Release and let go.

- *AHHHHH*. Expand, and expand further.

- Remain open and spacious.

- For the next 5 to 10 minutes, occasionally use the AH method to dissolve your awareness into space, like water being poured into water.

- At the conclusion, let go of any effort to meditate or breathe in any particular way and rest in silent stillness for a few minutes.

Practicing the Letting Go AH Practice in a formal med-itative session is deeply grounding. You might also use it spontaneously to regulate your nervous system throughout the day, weaving into your daily life the thread of memento mori and letting go.

KEY INSIGHTS

- Death is a constant reminder of what is most precious. *Memento mori—remember, I will die*—is a daily contemplation that all things pass, including ourselves. Contemplating death is the great priori-tizer and spurs us to love deeply.

- Letting go at the end of the exhale, pouring your awareness into space after the exhalation, is a preparation for when you take your last breath.

- Contemplating death might trigger anxiety; this is a natural response. Death anxiety is a signal for inquiry, offering insight. Use your breathing tool kit to navigate these feelings.

Chapter 13

BREATHING YOUR LAST BREATH

Why do we practice anything? To become competent, skilled, or even master a given activity, right?

To become adept at a skill, consistent and deliberate practice is essential. This has been the foundation of AIR—awareness, intervention, and regulation. It takes practice.

When you learned to drive a car, you didn't jump behind the wheel and head onto the freeway. Instead, you were mentored by your parents or an instructor, slowly and repeatedly driving around a parking lot or side streets, getting used to the steering wheel, brakes, gears, and your surroundings. The same goes for learning every activity that you are skilled at today, physical or mental. Just as you have progressively worked toward competency in breathing, the same goes for gaining skill in the last moment of our lives. We can practice breathing our last breath.

There is an ancient inscription carved above the entryway of the 10th-century St. Paul's Monastery on the secluded Mount Athos peninsula in Northern Greece. It reads: *If you die before you die, you won't die when you die.* This carries the profound message from memento mori to live life well, we must die before we die. We need to cathartically release our avoidance of the fact that we will die. There are a number of ways that ancients suggest we "die before we die" that include fasting, yoga and physical austerities, deep prayer, and meditation. During the Eleusinian mysteries, the Greeks would drink the psychoactive *kykeon* brew to enter non-ordinary states of consciousness where a metaphorical death occurred so they could be reborn to what is most essential and meaningful while still alive.[1]

Taking encouragement from the Greeks, as well as from the Buddhists, we'll now move into contemplating and meditating on our own death—to die before we die, so we don't have to die when we die. These practices are meant to be visceral. If you have read this far, you are most likely feeling prepared for death practices. Still, proceed slowly, perhaps just reading the words, as if you were studying them, and then when you feel ready, engage more fully in the meditation. If death anxiety arises, use your breath to regulate and calm your nervous system. Go slow. Be gentle with yourself. Feel deeply.

The first of our two death practices is the Nine Contemplations on Death, which is adapted from Tibetan Buddhist sources.‡‡‡‡ There isn't anything unique to Buddhism in the nine contemplations. Death is universal. The truth of death is not determined by any religious tradition or philosophical school. That said, this distillation of the

‡‡‡‡ The Nine Contemplations on Death are adapted from two sources in Tibet, Atisha Dipankara's 11th-century teachings and the legendary scholar-monk Jey Tsong Khapa's magnum opus from the 15th century, *The Great Treatise on the Stages of the Path to Enlightenment*. Jey Tsong Khapa's unique presentation of the nine contemplations drew from two principal sources: the famed 3rd-century Buddhist adept, Nagarjuna, in his *Letter to a King* and Atisha Dipankara's teachings. I was first taught The Nine Contemplation of Death in 1994 at Kopan Monastery in Nepal by the Swedish nun Ani Karin and Khenpo Konchok. I later studied the nine contemplations as well as the Death Rehearsal Meditation with Lama Zopa Rinpoche in Nepal, Chagdud Tulku Rinpoche in the U.S., and Geshe Tashi Tsering at Jamyang Buddhist Center in London.

Buddhists' vast teachings on death and impermanence into nine points for daily contemplation is as concise and impactful as you will find.

PRACTICE

Nine Contemplations on Death

Find a comfortable sitting position. Place your attention on the movement of your inhalation and exhalation for a few breaths to relax the body and mind.

Setting your intention, think: *Today I'm going to contemplate death so that I may live life to its fullest extent.*

The first contemplation: *Death is certain.* Everyone who is born must die. I'm not special. Nobody escapes death. What am I doing right now to live life fully and that will help me die without regrets?

The second contemplation: *My life span is always decreasing.* Each breath brings me closer to death. Every day my days are fewer. Because I'm getting closer to death, what am I doing today to contribute to a tranquil passing? Have I told my family and friends today how much I love and appreciate them?

The third contemplation: *Death comes whether or not I'm prepared.* Everyone dies, no matter how privileged or wealthy. Am I speaking to others in my life like it is the last time I will see them?

Conviction: *Because death is certain, I seize the opportunity today to fully develop my potential and positive mental qualities.*

The fourth contemplation: *The time of my death is uncertain.* How many people died today who did not expect to? I might die this evening; there is no guarantee. I might die in my sleep. How can I live today like it is my last? When I die, will I have any regrets?

The fifth contemplation: *Death has many causes.* There are innumerable ways to die. I can die today from an accident. Deadly sickness is a real possibility. How can I prepare my mind and heart so that I die without regrets?

The sixth contemplation: *My human body is fragile and vulnerable.* When I exhale, there is no guarantee I'll inhale. My life hangs on each breath. There's no guarantee I won't have a heart attack or stroke today. Do my body's aches and pains remind me that they will soon give way totally? Am I using my body to show love to my family and others?

Conviction: *Because the time of death is uncertain, I won't delay in developing my full potential and positive mental qualities.*

The seventh contemplation: *At the time of death, my possessions and wealth are of no use.* No physical possessions that I've worked so hard for in my life matter at the time of death. Money is useless at death. As I look around my home, how many things do I see that will end up thrown away or at the thrift store? I may have some attachments to my material wealth as I die, so better I give them away before so that my mind is untethered. How can I release my attachment to physical possessions today?

The eighth contemplation: *My loved ones cannot keep me from death. There is no delaying its advent.* No matter how much my family loves me, they can do nothing for me when death comes. If the people I hold most dear can't do anything for me at the time of death, how am I preparing?

The ninth contemplation: *My body cannot help me at the time of death. I must let go.* I have put so much effort into taking care of this body for so long with amazing food, lotions and creams, soft and protective clothing, and perfumes and colognes. How much time have I spent preparing my mind for death? I've tried to make my body always look younger, more attractive, and hang on to its youthful vigor, but in the end, it will dry up and die. Will my body be cremated or eaten by worms after it's buried? When I die, can I let go of this physical body that I have spent so many years caring for? Isn't it better to use my abilities today to benefit my family and community?

Conviction: *The only help I'll have at the time of death is the strength of my mind and positive mental qualities.*

Conclusion of meditation: These Nine Contemplations on Death prepare me to meet my death without regret. Death is certain, the timing is uncertain, and I take responsibility for my state of mind and heart right now. Death is never easy. When death comes, I'll let go and surrender, not holding on to my body, my possessions, and especially my thoughts. Starting today, I renew my commitment to preparing my mind for my death by strengthening my capacity to let go and surrender.

You can move through all nine in a single session, spending a few minutes on each contemplation. Or, if you want to take one contemplation and use it as a memento mori touchstone for a day or a week, that can also be effective. The point is to imbue your awareness and be with the truth of your mortality.

Create Your Own Reminders of Memento Mori

Throughout the centuries, artists and philosophers have created their own meaningful reminders of impermanence, of our mortality. These have included the classic paintings and sculptures with the *Vanitas* motifs of a skull (death), wilting flowers (life), and an hourglass (time). I encourage you to find an image that pierces through the intellect and stirs your heart as a memento mori reminder. I use an image of a skeleton of rib bones and sternum with beautiful flowers as my daily reminder. You might display your own insights or the words of others, like the poet Lisel Mueller (who fled the Nazi regime at age 15), who wrote in *In Passing*, "as if what exists, exists/so that it can be lost/and become precious" or as Roman emperor and Stoic philosopher Marcus Aurelius advised, "Let each thing you would do, say, or intend be like that of a dying person."[2]

As you practice memento mori, the constant changes of life around you emerge in greater clarity. There is less solidity and more flow; less grasping and more allowing. In that realization of impermanence around you, you might find:

- The end of every exhale is a reminder that you are closer to death—*let go of any regrets.*

- Sunrises and sunsets, the beginning and end of each day, remind you of the transient nature of life and inevitability of death—*tell a loved one how much you care for them.*

- Falling leaves that started as a budding leaf opened, fluttered, and then fell off the tree remind you of the cycle of birth, growth, and death—*find joy in the small pleasures.*

- Every single thing you do today may be for the last time—*seize this day with enthusiasm.*

- Aches and pains are the natural aging process that leads to death—*don't put off telling your family that you love them.*

- Seasons are continually changing, from the vibrant growth of spring that transitions to the dormant stillness of winter, reminding you of the arising and passing of all things— *let this remind you to generate gratitude for what you have.*

- Natural disasters like earthquakes, hurricanes, and wildfires remind you of the fragility of life and suddenness with which it can be taken away—*there are no guarantees in life so express your joy today.*

- The stages of your child's growth, especially when they leave home, remind you of constant change—*be fully present with what is before you now, not what is no longer.*

- Shadows accompany you wherever you go, so too does the inevitability of death—*remember memento mori.*

Regularly contemplating death and practicing memento mori may stir the question within us: *Can I prepare for when I actually die?* This question leads to the next practice of rehearsing our own death. The point of rehearsing death is to become so familiar with the process of dying that it doesn't distract you from resting in the awareness of the unfolding of the experience. This is no doubt a tall order because life, your life, is literally extinguishing itself, dissolving around you.

Death Is a Process

We often think that death is when our vital organs, principally our heart or brain, stop. Yet death doesn't happen in a single moment; it's a process. Current medical studies show that your awareness does not cease immediately when your body, or even your brain, ceases to function. Research on near-death experiences in the last two decades records numerous occasions when individuals who have been deemed clinically dead by a medical professional have accurately reported events that occurred around them, at home and in the hospital or surgery unit. The connection between perception and brain activity is not totally understood, but the research on near-death experiences indicates that consciousness may continue for minutes after breathing and cardiac function ends. Tibetan Buddhism teaches that it can be days after the breath ceases before the death process concludes.

By contemplating death like the ancients have encouraged while reading the current scientific research, it is hard not to recognize how extraordinarily unique the experience of dying is. There is an exquisiteness, it seems, to be lucidly aware, free of anxiety, as the last breath is taken before entering the portal of death, and the journey beyond, if there is one. Of course, the timing of our death is uncertain, and if it is accidental or happens suddenly, then the dying process may be so quick that there is little time to draw upon past contemplative experience. But even in the case of a sudden death, such as a heart attack, recent studies indicate that you may become hyperalert at the time of death because of a surge of electricity to the brain.[3]

Practicing Dying

The Death Rehearsal Meditation below originates from the same Buddhist tradition that produced the Nine

Contemplations of Death. It is a practice that has been adopted by hospice workers and palliative care providers in non-Buddhist situations because it provides solace and anxiety relief for not only the dying person but also their loved ones and caregivers. The physiological indicators during the dying process, such as the progressive fading of physical senses, change in skin tone, the sound of the death rattle, and other signposts, are meditated upon so that we become familiar with the process.[4] This Death Rehearsal Meditation requires no belief or dogmatic adherences.

In this death practice, you are simulating dying. You imagine and visualize the gradual shutting down of the functions of your body related to the four elements of earth, water, fire, and air, as well as the fading of your five senses of seeing, hearing, smelling, touching, and tasting. This is called the outer dissolution—your physical form is dying. Every single one of us will experience this.

Then the inner dissolution follows when the constituents of your mind—feelings, perceptions, and intellect—progressively exhaust themselves, dissolving into the most subtle aspects of your consciousness before finally leaving the body. During the meditation, which is meant to be memorized, you train to recognize death's external and especially internal signs, such as the visionary experiences. Familiarity of these signs help us continually let go into the experience of dying when it actually happens. This is why we are practicing dying, so we are prepared when it happens.

As you move through the dissolution of "you" and everything you experience, the main practice is releasing and letting go. We've practiced various ways to let go earlier in this book, especially connected to our exhale, and those pulmonautic skills are applied here. The sense of who you are right now, all your associated identities, personality, and roles, you are now letting go and releasing that into spaciousness, into vastness. By releasing the elements of your identity that compose what you know as "I" and "me," you are releasing your body and all the patterns and habits in the mind. Contemplating this, imagining this happening, is not easy, but it is part of dying well.

The death process is the progressive dissolution of the body and mind until the essence of your being, your consciousness, leaves the body. There are different names for this essence—you might call it your soul, spirt, atman, essence, or being. In the practice below, I call this essence *consciousness*, but feel free to associate that with whatever you hold and name to be your essence.

Proceed cautiously—this meditation may evoke strong emotional responses, including death anxiety. Use the breath as needed to navigate strong emotions. This practice is suitable for everyone except those who experience suicidal ideation or have mental health conditions including anxiety disorders or posttraumatic stress disorder.

PRACTICE

Death Rehearsal Meditation

During this meditation, imagine you are dying. Notice what happens in your mind and body. Emotions, visual images, and reactions to the idea of dying may arise during this Death Rehearsal Meditation—that is part of the reason to do this practice. Allow emotions and feelings to rise, be noticed, pass through your mind and body, and then be released. There is no need to hang on to or to push back against any feelings or emotions.

This practice is about awakening to your essential spaciousness, so release and let go. Rehearsing your death takes courage. There is nothing to be afraid of. Use your breath during the practice to relax deeper and deeper. Extend your exhales to help the releasing and letting go—this is applied not only during this meditation but also when you die. You are practicing breathing your last breaths.

Posture and Motivation

Find a comfortable seated position. Or you can assume the auspicious posture known as the "sleeping lion position," the posture that the Buddha was in when he died. Lie on your right side, knees slightly drawn up. Your left arm rests along your left side. Your right hand supports your head with your hand holding your cheek. If you like, lightly press your little finger against your right nostril so that you breathe only through your left nostril, stimulating your parasympathetic nervous system.

If you find meaning and solace in an image of Jesus, Mother Mary, the Buddha, Shiva, Abraham, or another being who represents to you the essence of love, compassion, and awakening, point the crown of your head toward that blessed image.

Gently close your eyes. Or, if you like, leave your eyes partially open so that you don't create a duality between inside and outside. There is no need to pay special attention to either the inside or the outside, but simply withdraw your attention away from your visual stimulation to rest in your mental landscape. Let your eyes be still and not darting here and there.

Begin to settle the body and mind with breath awareness for a few moments. If you become distracted during this practice, release the thinking, relax completely, and return to the breath for a few moments. Continually release, relax, and return to the breath.

If you find that strong emotions arise during the practice, there is no need to block them or hold on to them. Allow them to move through your awareness. Extending your exhale, breathe with the emotions.

Before you begin your Death Rehearsal Meditation, think: *Whatever insights come from my meditation today, may they not only benefit myself, but also my family, my community, and beyond.*

The Outer Dissolution of Your Senses

Imagine you are dying. You are in your bed at home or hospital. Your family and friends are around you. Your sight is waning, and you can't make out who's who in the room. Your family is speaking, but you don't understand. You can't taste or smell any longer. Your ability to feel anything on your skin is fading. You are confused as your five physical senses begin to dissolve. Let go of any agitation in your mind. Release. Let go. This is a sign the dying process has started. You are dying.

THE OUTER DISSOLUTION OF THE EARTH ELEMENT INTO WATER ELEMENT

Your Form Is Dissolving

Your body will soon unbind itself. You can't sit up, raise your hand, or hold your head up. You have no energy. Let go and allow your body to die. There is a sense of falling or being pushed down. Your body is becoming heavier. It's as if a great weight is pressing your shoulders down, your sternum down, your hips down into the bed. The dense heaviness is uncomfortable, and you might try to motion to change positions. Your skin is pale as your blood circulation is slowing. Your heartbeat is faint.

The earth element becomes weaker. The form of our body is coming apart, dissolving, becoming weak and frail. Your relationship to the physical world is no longer. Heaviness, drowsiness, being pushed down, your inability to see the world of form; this is you dying. Let go. Remain present. Don't be frightened. Release. Witness the physical body dying. This body is not you.

Visions begin to swirl in your mind like shimmering blue mirages. You don't see them with your eyes, they are behind your eyes. You feel like you are melting. This is the sign that the earth element is dissolving into water.

OUTER DISSOLUTION OF THE WATER ELEMENT INTO FIRE ELEMENT

Your Ability to Feel Is Dissolving

Your body is drying up. You are losing control of bodily fluids. Drool comes out the side of your mouth, your nose is running, and you can't hold your urine. Your skin is cold to touch and feels papery. Your lips crack, and the tongue feels like it swells in the back of your throat. Your nostrils collapse, and you're thirsty. Let go of the need to drink anything. You are dying. When you blink, your eyes feel scratchy and sting. Do not be afraid. The water element in your body is dissolving into the fire element.

The water element becomes weaker. Your ability to feel sensation is waning, but still there are passing experiences of being hot and cold, brief waves of pleasure and pain. If you feel upset or agitated, try to let go. You are dying. The body is drying up. Sounds your family make in the room are like distant echoes. You have no energy to concentrate. Remain present. Don't be frightened. Release. Allow your mind to witness the body dying. This body is not you.

Everything seems to be smoky around you. This is an internal vision. This is the sign the water element is dissolving into fire element.

OUTER DISSOLUTION OF THE FIRE ELEMENT INTO AIR ELEMENT

Your Perception Is Dissolving

The fire element in your body is dissolving into air. Your mouth, nose, and eyes have no moisture. Your body feels cool as any warmth in the body moves toward your heart. Your hands and feet are cold. The little breath that remains is cold. Your inhale may be short and weak while your exhale may become like a long sigh.

The fire element becomes weaker. Your consciousness moves between inner lucidity and hallucinations. You can't perceive the outer world around you any longer. Your faculties to see, hear, taste, feel, or smell no longer function. Perceptions based upon forms and feeling have ceased. You've lost the ability to remember the name of your family. Your experience is mostly internal. Remain present. Don't be frightened. Release. Allow your experience to unfold. You are dying.

The smoky visions in your mind have morphed into a vision of sparks throughout the universe. It is as if millions of blue-green fireflies are swirling around your entire being. This is a sign that the fire element has dissolved into the air element.

OUTER DISSOLUTION OF THE AIR ELEMENT INTO CONSCIOUSNESS

Your Intellect Is Dissolving

The air element is dissolving into your consciousness. Some saliva might pool in the back of your throat and make a rattling sound. Your eyes have rolled up into your skull or gaze empty outward. Halting, uneven breaths may come, or you may pant. You are no longer aware of your own breath, or who is in the room. Your last experiences of the outer world are finishing. There's nothing to do. Do not be afraid as your dying continues.

The air element becomes weaker. Your inner visions are increasing. Let go completely. The visions that arise come from who you are and how you have lived. The visions are reflections of past experiences— but they are just visions. You might not understand what appears—relax and let go. Family and ancestors might appear—allow the vision to unfold without grasping, let go. Teachers or saints or friends may offer messages—allow the vision to unfold without holding on to them. Intensely emotional events from your life may surface—release and let go. You may meet threatening, dangerous, or scary visions as if you are in hell—they are visions. Let them go. If you have harmed people or animals during your life, they may appear in visions—you are dying; let go of the visions. Whatever visions arise, there is no need to identify with them. You are dying.

The images from your past begin to decrease. Your body feels no sensations. Thoughts and thinking have ceased. Breathing has stopped. Brain waves have stopped. Your family sees you as dead. Feel the stillness. Melt into this empty state. Become vast emptiness. Any

remaining energy of your life has dissolved into consciousness at your heart. Your chest is slightly warm.

When you have an internal vision of a small,
flickering flame, like a candle in the wind, this is the
moment of your physical death. This is the sign the air
element has dissolved into the most subtle level of your
consciousness at your heart. Let go.

THE INNER DISSOLUTION

Consciousness Departs the Body

The vision of the flickering light slowly diminishes.
Do not be afraid. Consciousness will depart the body
after the most subtle levels of the mind dissolve.

The essence of the energy you received from
your father is in the form of a white energy-drop and
descends from your crown along the spine toward your
consciousness at your heart. With great clarity, you
experience an all-encompassing vision of moonlight.

Then, the essence you received from your mother
in the form of a red energy-drop ascends along the
spine from just below the navel toward the heart,
bringing an experience of great bliss. You experience a
vision of all-compassing red sunlight.

When the white and red energy-drops meet at
the heart, they encase your consciousness, and for a
moment, utter darkness is experienced like a black sky
with no light. You experience blank vacuity, unconscious. Do not fear. Let go.

From the momentary darkness, the clear light of
death begins to dawn like an immaculate, crystalline
sky, free of clouds or mist. Everything is transparent.
You are one with a clear dawn sky, free of moonlight,

sunlight, and darkness. This luminous clear light is the source of consciousness, completely pure and unstained. Expand and abide in the primordial ground of being.

Allow your crystal-clear consciousness to exit from the top of your head through the fontanel and mingle in unconfined space. Boundless. Free.

Rest here for however long thought-free awareness remains.

Conclusion of Meditation

Let go of the visualization and rest the mind for a few minutes. And then think for a moment: *May my effort at rehearsing my death prepare me for dying without regret.*

How Long Does the Natural Death Process Take?

You might wonder how long the outer and inner dissolution takes before your consciousness departs the body. That is to say, how long does it take to die? There are different circumstances, but from the time you start to experience diminishing of the five senses coupled with the inner smoke-like vision, according to Tibetan Buddhist teachings, it takes anywhere from minutes to three days for the death process to exhaust itself. This is the reason it is ideal not to disturb the body for a few days after the person has stopped breathing.

Until the end of the outer dissolution, your mind still functions, even though you may not be engaged with the outer world. Awareness is heightened, and you can be easily affected by the environment around you, including what others do, say, and think. In your advanced directive or living will, you may ask to keep the environment very calm and peaceful without the presence of televisions, radio, and other discursive noises. You can also have in your directive to ask that a spiritual friend or family member gently remind you of the positive aspects of your life, the unconditional love of your family, or whatever other messages that are supportive. In the early stages, it might be helpful to be reminded to gently focus on your breathing, to let go of your body and the outer world, and that you are dying.

During the inner dissolution when your mind is extinguishing itself before your consciousness departs the body, it's recommended that your body not be disturbed, as if you were in deep sleep. If there is a reason to move your body before the dying process is complete, it is recommended that a spiritual friend or family member tap the crown of the head or slightly tug on the hair at the crown to encourage your consciousness to exit from this portal.

Advance Directive

As a natural progression from the Nine Contemplations on Death and the Death Rehearsal Meditation, it's common to think about actionable preparations for our end-of-life scenarios. One highly practical step that harmonizes with death and dying practices is creating an advance directive, also called a living will. With your advance directive, you designate a trusted individual to make decisions on your behalf when you are no longer able to do so, including guidance to your loved ones regarding the extent of medical interventions, pain management, and life-sustaining support you desire. An advance directive is an integral part of the art of letting go. It enables you to free yourself from the weight of decision-making and apprehension, allowing you to focus on what truly matters.

Recognizing that this is a deeply personal decision, approach the process with tenderness, acknowledging that articulating your wishes may bring a profound sense of peace and comfort but also sadness. It may even evoke emotions similar to death anxiety. Taking the time to reflect on and clearly express your preferences enables your family and friends to focus on providing support, love, and understanding as you approach your final moments, knowing that your choices have lightened their burden of decision making.

Establishing your advance directive costs little or is free. Documents and processes vary by state and country, so ask your family doctor, lawyer, healthcare worker, or aging and end-of-life organizations for more information as needed.

Beyond Death

What happens after death? I have no experience, so I cannot say definitively. I know that any belief I have is an opinion, and I keep in mind what Leonardo Da Vinci cautioned, when he said, "The greatest deception men suffer is from their own opinions." My own near-death experience when the tree fell on me only took me in front of the door that leads to the beyond. I only knocked at death's doorstep and did not venture far into the dissolution process before returning to tend to my wounds. Near-death experiences are just that: near.

Beliefs about what happens after death vary greatly among individuals and cultures. I know many religious or spiritual teachers who purport to know and what various scriptures and holy books tell us about what happens after death. Nearly everyone I ask responds with some story about what lies beyond death, even for those who believe it is utter annihilation or a "nothingness." While some people hold firm beliefs about the nature of an afterlife, such as heaven, hell, reincarnation, or spiritual continuation, others may view it as an unknown or unknowable aspect of existence. Our story of what is beyond death is shaped by personal experiences, cultural, religious, or philosophical backgrounds, and individual interpretations. These beliefs are very important and offer solace when we are dying.

All my Buddhist teachers believe in reincarnation and have a lot to teach about what happens after death, which is why they say, "The next breath or the next life—which will come first is uncertain." Still, with sincere respect to my teachers, I return to the Buddha's injunction to rely on the truth of one's own experience rather than faith alone. When I consider what is beyond death, I contemplate the act of lighting one candle with another and ask myself, *Are the two flames the same or different?*

Living without Regrets

Whatever happens after death, dying peacefully and without regrets is the reason to practice dying, to become familiar right now with breathing your last breath. We can take encouragement from Frank Ostaseski's words: "Harness the awareness of death to appreciate the fact that we are alive, to encourage self-exploration, to clarify our values, to find meaning, and to generate positive action. It is the impermanence of life that gives us perspective. As we come in contact with life's precarious nature, we also come to appreciate its preciousness. Then we don't want to waste a minute. We want to enter our lives fully and use them in a responsible way. Death is a good companion on the road to living well and dying without regret."[5]

You can't predict when your last breath will be. But in this moment, you have the power to choose how to live. We forgive and ask for forgiveness, including of ourselves. Embracing the truth of our ephemeral existence and mortality daily, a natural sorting out of what is truly important in your life emerges with precision. It illuminates the insignificance of our fleeting angers, blames, and resentments, urging us to leave a lasting impact of joy and sweetness that the world can cherish. Memento mori is a reminder to take full responsibility for your mind and heart, to give and receive love, while you are alive so that there will be no regrets when your last exhalation comes. As Viktor Frankl wrote in *Yes to Life: In Spite of Everything*, "As long as we have breath, as long as we are still conscious, we are each responsible for answering life's questions. This should not surprise us once we recall the great fundamental truth of being human— being human is nothing other than being conscious and being responsible!"[6]

KEY INSIGHTS

- Meditating on our death awakens us to the most fundamental truth of existence—that all things pass. This bone-deep realization ignites a passion to live and love without reservation so that we die without regrets.

- All that we experience and have in life exists, and then passes, so that its preciousness can be known.

- Release and let go—this is the practice for today, and this is the practice for when you exhale your final breath.

Chapter 14

EACH BREATH IS AN OPPORTUNITY TO BEGIN AGAIN

When I began studying meditation some 30 years ago, I regularly went on extended retreats, sometimes in a group and other times alone. On my first monthlong meditation retreat, I was at a monastery on the outskirts of Kathmandu. Before sunrise, a handful of us gathered in a small chapel, wrapped in woolen blankets, sandalwood incense burning on the shrine before an inspiring image of the Buddha: the perfect conditions for a calm and concentrated meditation practice. Yet, even after weeks of meditating day and night, I found myself thinking about snowboarding back home, nice pasta meals in Rome, or composing letters in my mind to my family and friends. Concentration was elusive.

Anyone who has ever practiced meditation has experienced distraction, usually within a few moments of turning their attention inward. When we concentrate on an object, such as the breath, it is natural that the mind wanders away. We are all distractible; it's the human condition. Thoughts are alluring, and not only the nice ones. Thoughts of things we dislike or that annoy us still entice us to grasp them, mull over them, repeatedly think about them. This begins cycles of thinking about something in the future or something that happened in the past. When we catch ourselves thinking during meditation, often we don't know how long we've been distracted. It takes concentration training to rest in the ever-changing flow of experience that we call the present—this is one of the skills cultivated in meditation practice. But even for individuals who have mastered concentration practices, they will tell you that distraction is only a moment away.

A kind nun was overseeing that first meditation retreat—Ani Karin, the same nun who first taught me to contemplate death. Though we were in silence for the month, if we had questions, we could meet her in the evening to discuss. I decided to tell her about my dismay at how distracted my mind was. I fancied myself as a yogi in the Himalayas but continuous thoughts of snowboarding and eating fine food constantly diverted my attention! I felt defeated.

Ani Karin encouraged me to be kind to myself and not berate myself for being distracted. When I recognized I was distracted in meditation, she instructed, release the thinking, relax the body, and return attention to the breath. In this way, the so-called distracting thoughts themselves become a reminder to come back to the practice. Each time, release, relax, and return. "Each breath is an opportunity to begin again," she'd say.

The advice to continually "begin again" from over three decades ago has remained with me, not just in meditation practice but as advice for living. When we realize that each breath is an opportunity to begin again, it is as if a doorway to unlimited possibilities opens. This day, this hour, this minute, this very breath is pure potential.

And what do we find when we walk through that doorway of pure potentiality? As the Roman philosopher Cicero said, "Dum spiro, spero." As I breathe, I hope.

Breath is life. I learned this when the tree that was pinning me to the ground and suffocating me was lifted. Breath and life whooshed in simultaneously. Our breath is filled with potential and with our spirit. Breathing is inspiration. Each breath is an opportunity to begin again.

When we recognize at a fundamental level that our life and that of every individual around us is literally hanging on a breath, we see that we are all in the same boat. This recognition of the precarious, yet beautiful, predicament we are all in gives rise to kindness and a softening in our hearts toward ourselves and others. This kindness is the basis of hope that Cicero spoke of.

Paying attention to our breath is a profound way to connect to this hopefulness and a feeling to share it with others. The French philosopher and mystic Simone Weil wrote, "Attention is the rarest and purest form of generosity."[1] Attending to and directing our breath for our health and well-being is an act of generosity because we can then more effectively care for those whom we love. This is the power of our attentive awareness and the breath; that it can transform into acts of generosity.

We started our breath journey in this book with AIR—awareness of the breath, initiation of breathing interventions, and regulation of our nervous system. Whether we recognized it at the time or not, we were optimizing the breath to breathe how we want to feel, and AIR is also about having the energy and capacity to care for those around us and for the causes we want to advance. This is why there was a brief motivation in all the guided practices in this book to remind us that we are here to serve others. Suffusing our mind and breath with this sense of hopefulness and generosity opens our heart to gratitude.

The following practice is to grow this sense of gratitude for our breath, for our being, and to connect to others.

PRACTICE

Gratitude for My Breath, Gratitude for My Time

Find a comfortable position, gently close your eyes, and take a few deep breaths to settle into the present moment.

Contemplate for a moment: *Thankful for my breath and for the inspiration it brings me, I commit to serving my family and my community. As we embark on this gratitude meditation, I'm cultivating appreciation for my breath, the time I have left to live, and the kindness shown by others.*

Take a slow, long breath and feel a sense of gratitude welling up within you for your own strength, resilience, and inherent goodness.

Gratitude for the Breath
Keep your awareness on your breath, your constant companion that accompanies you in every moment. Take a moment to appreciate the simple yet profound gift of breath, the life force that nourishes your body and sustains you. Breathe however you feel nourishes you.

With each inhale, feel the life-giving energy entering your body.

With each exhale, let go of any tension or stress.

Offer gratitude for the innate wisdom of your body, effortlessly and rhythmically breathing, keeping you alive and allowing you to love and be loved.

Gratitude for the Time We Have Remaining

Reflect on the preciousness of the time you have remaining. You know the preciousness of things because they will not be here forever.

Breathe in this moment with immense gratitude for life.

Breathe out that which does not serve you any longer.

Breath in and feel gratitude for the time you have left to live, no matter how long or short it may be.

Breathe out and let go.

Embrace the truth that each day holds the potential for growth, joy, and meaningful connections. Recognize that this very moment is a gift.

With gratitude, commit to making the most of the time you have, living fully and authentically.

Gratitude for the Kindness of Others

Shift your attention to the kindness shown to you by others in your life.

Think of those close to you, or animals, who have extended love and support your way. Feel their love.

Breathe in the affection and love they have shown you.

Breathe out and allow that love to pervade your entire being.

Offer gratitude for the teachers, mentors, and role models who have shared their wisdom and insights with you. Recognize the impact they have had on your personal and spiritual development, and how they continue to shape your path.

Breathe in their wisdom.

Breathe out and allow that wisdom to spread in your heart and mind.

Allow a sense of gratitude to arise for the connections that exists with your family, friends, and community. Take a moment to silently express your gratitude for their presence in your life and the small and larger ways they've influenced you.

Breathe in the love they give you.

Breathe out love to your family and community.

Conclusion

Gently bring your awareness back to your breath.

Feel your nourishing breath.

Inhale gratitude with a smile.

Exhale and let go completely.

Let gratitude's warmth fill your entire being.

When you're ready, open your eyes, returning to the present moment, and greet the world with a heart full of gratitude.

My Hope for Your Journey

As you have journeyed through this book, my sincere hope is that you have gained knowledge and an experiential understanding of the profound power that lies within your breath. May you continue to explore with a childlike curiosity the vast potential that each inhale and exhale carries. When you fully grasp the transformative nature of your breath, it becomes a dynamic force that moves through every fiber of your being, touching your mind, body, and spirit.

As you cultivate a harmonious relationship with your breath, may the benefits extend far beyond your individual experience and bring you into deeper connection with your loved ones and the world. Together, let us embrace the potential that lies within each breath and breathe in the fullness of life itself.

Know that you are not alone on this journey of breath. In our shared exploration, may you find inspiration, guidance, and friends to navigate the intricacies of life. As you continue on this path, may your breath remain a trusted companion, guiding you toward a life that is not only vibrant and fulfilling but also aligned with your deepest intentions and aspirations.

And let us always remember that it is the breath that weaves together the threads of life, connecting you, me, our families, and our communities. Everything that breathes is filled with life. With each inhalation, we draw in the essence of existence, infusing our being with vitality. And as we exhale, our spirit generously gives back, showering the world with the life-giving breath. It is this sacred rhythm of breath, the cosmic pulse of inhalations and exhalations, that unites all living beings.

The air you inhale transforms into the life-sustaining breath that animates your very being. And the breath you exhale becomes air that I and everyone inhale that nourishes us. Let us cherish this precious reciprocity, for in every breath, we are reminded of our shared journey. May we embrace the oneness that flows through every living entity, nourishing our hearts and souls with a profound sense of interconnectedness.

ENDNOTES

Introduction: Breath Is Life

1. David Garrigues, *Vayu Siddhi: A Guide to Pranayama, Ashtanga Yoga's Fourth Limb* (Philadelphia: BookBaby, 2015).

2. Balban et al., "Brief Structured Respiration Practices Enhance Mood and Reduce Physiological Arousal," *Cell Reports Medicine* 4, no. 1 (2023): 100895, doi:10.1016/j.xcrm.2022.100895z.

Chapter 1: Breath Is the Most Fundamental Aspect of Your Being

1. Kiesel et al., "Development of a Screening Protocol to Identify Individuals with Dysfunctional Breathing," *International Journal of Sports Physical Therapy* 12, no. 5 (October 2017): 774–786.

2. Peter Attia, *Outlive: The Science and Art of Longevity* (New York: Harmony, 2023).

3. Fincham et al., "Effect of Breathwork on Stress and Mental Health: A Meta-Analysis of Randomised-Controlled Trials," *Scientific Reports* 13, (2023): 432, https://doi.org/10.1038/s41598-022-27247-y.

4. Torah: Job 33:4 (Koren Jerusalem Bible); Bible: Genesis 2:7 (New International Version); Koran: 15:28-29 (Surah-Al Hijr).

5. Bible: John 20:19-22 (NIV).

6. *The Bhagavadgītā in the Mahābhārata* (trans. and ed. J. A. B. van Buitenen), (London/Chicago: The University of Chicago Press, 1981). *The Hatha Yoga Pradipika: The Original Sanskrit by Svatmarama* (trans. Brian Dana Ackers) (Woodstock, NY: YogaVidya.com, 2002). Pradeep P. Gokhale, *The Yogasūtra of Patañjali: A New Introduction to the Buddhist Roots of the Yoga System* (India: Taylor & Francis, 2020). James Mallinson and Mark Singleton, *Roots of Yoga* (New York: Penguin Books, 2017). Mark Singleton, *Yoga Body: The Origins of Modern Posture Practice* (Oxford/New York: Oxford University Press, 2010).

7. James Mallinson, *The Amṛtasiddhi and Amṛtasiddhimūla—The Earliest Texts of the Haṭhayoga Tradition* (Pondichery, India: Institut Francais De Pondichery, 2021).

8. Dr. Andrew Weil, *Breathing: The Master Key to Self-Healing* (Boulder, Colo.: Sounds True, 2001).

Chapter 2: Cultivating Awareness

1. Elissa Epel, Ph.D., *The Stress Prescription: 7 Days to More Joy and Ease* (New York: Penguin Books, 2022).

2. Philippot, Chapelle, and Blairy, "Respiratory Feedback in the Generation of Emotion," *Cognition and Emotion* 16 no. 5 (September 10, 2015): 605–627, doi: 10.1080/02699930143000392.

3. Harrison et al., "Interoception of breathing and its relationship with anxiety," *Neuron* 109, no. 24 (December 2021): 4080–4093.e8, https://doi.org/10.1016/j.neuron.2021.09.045.

Chapter 3: Adjusting the Dials on Your Nervous System

1. Elissa Epel, Ph.D., *The Stress Prescription: 7 Days to More Joy and Ease* (New York: Penguin Books, 2022).

2. Kox et al., "Voluntary Activation of the Sympathetic Nervous System and Attenuation of the Innate Immune Response in Humans," *Proceedings of the National Academy of Sciences* 111, no. 20 (May 2014): 7379–84, doi: 10.1073/pnas.1322174111.

3. Curley, Kavanagh, and Laffey, "Hypocapnia and the Injured Brain: Evidence for Harm," *Critical Care Medicine* 39, no. 1 (2011): 229–230, https://doi.org/10.1097/CCM.0b013e3181ffe3c7. Kane et al., "Hyperventilation During Electroencephalography: Safety and Efficacy," *Seizure* 23, no. 2 (2014): 129–134, https://doi.org/10.1016/j.seizure.2013.10.010. King et al., "Failure of Perception of Hypocapnia: Physiological and Clinical Implications," *Journal of the Royal Society of Medicine* 83, no.12 (1990): 765–767, https://doi.org/10.1177/014107689008301205.

4. Bernardi et al., "Effect of Rosary Prayer and Yoga Mantras on Autonomic Cardiovascular Rhythms: Comparative Study," *BMJ* 323, no. 7327 (December 22–29, 2001): 1446–9, doi: 10.1136/bmj.323.7327.1446.

5. Zaccaro et al., "Neural Correlates of Non-Ordinary States of Consciousness in Pranayama Practitioners: The Role of Slow Nasal Breathing," *Frontiers in Systems Neuroscience* 16 (March 21, 2022): 803904, doi: 10.3389/fnsys.2022.803904.

Chapter 4: Breathing through Your Nose

1. James Nestor, *Breath: The New Science of a Lost Art* (New York: Riverhead Books, 2020).

2. Lundberg et al., "Inhalation of Nasally Derived Nitric Oxide Modulates Pulmonary Function in Humans," *Acta Physiologica Scandanavia* 158, no. 4 (December 1996): 343–7, doi: 10.1046/j.1365-201X.1996.557321000.x.

3. Sanchez et al., "Nasal Nitric Oxide and Regulation of Human Pulmonary Blood Flow in the Upright Position," *Journal of Applied Physiology* 108 (2010): 181–188, doi: 10.1152/japplphysiol.00285.2009.

4. Lundberg and Weitzberg, "Nasal Nitric Oxide in Man," *Thorax* 54, no. 10 (1999): 947–952, https://doi.org/10.1136/thx.54.10.947. Bath et al., "Nitric Oxide for the Prevention and Treatment of Viral, Bacterial, Protozoal and Fungal Infections," *F1000Research* 10, no. 536 (2021), https://doi.org/10.12688/f1000research.51270.2.

5. Zaccaro et al., "How Breath-Control Can Change Your Life: A Systematic Review on Psycho-Physiological Correlates of Slow Breathing," *Frontiers in Human Neuroscience* 12 (September 2018): 353, doi: 10.3389/fnhum.2018.00353. Laborde et al., "Effects of Voluntary Slow Breathing on Heart Rate and Heart Rate Variability: A Systematic Review and Meta-Analysis," *Neuroscience and Biobehavior Reviews* 138 (July 2022): 104711, doi: 10.1016/j.neubiorev.2022.104711.

6. Stephen Porges, *The Polyvagal Theory: Neurophysiological Foundations of Emotions, Attachment, Communication, and Self-regulation* (New York: W. W. Norton & Company, 2011).

7. Gerritsen and Band, "Breath of Life: The Respiratory Vagal Stimulation Model of Contemplative Activity," *Frontiers in Human Neuroscience* 12 (October 2018): 397, doi: 10.3389/fnhum.2018.00397.

8. Kalyani et al., "Neurohemodynamic Correlates of 'OM' Chanting: A Pilot Functional Magnetic Resonance Imaging Study," *International Journal of Yoga* 4, no. 1 (January 2011): 3–6. doi: 10.4103/0973-6131.78171.

9. Eby, "Strong Humming for One Hour Daily to Terminate Chronic Rhinosinusitis in Four Days: A Case Report and Hypothesis for Action by Stimulation of Endogenous Nasal Nitric Oxide Production," *Medical Hypotheses* 66, no. 4 (2006): 851–4, doi: 10.1016/j.mehy.2005.11.035.

10. Lundberg et al., "Humming, Nitric Oxide, and Paranasal Sinus Obstruction," *Journal of the American Medical Association* 289, no. 3 (January 2003): 302–3, doi: 10.1001/jama.289.3.302-b.

11. Kuppusamy et al., "Effects of *Bhramari Pranayama* on Health—A Systematic Review," *Journal of Traditional and Complementary Medicine* 8, no. 1 (March 2017): 11–16, doi: 10.1016/j.jtcme .2017.02.003.

12. Lunn and Craig, "Rhinitis and Sleep," *Sleep Medicine Reviews* 15, no. 5 (October 2011): 293–9. Muliol, Maurer, and Bousquet, "Sleep and Allergic Rhinitis," *Journal of Investigation Allergology Clinical Immunology* 18, no. 6 (2008): 415–9. Ohki et al., "Relationship Between Oral Breathing and Nasal Obstruction in Patients with Obstructive Sleep Apnoea," *Acta Oto-Laryngologica Supplement* 523 (1996): 228–30. Fried, in (eds.) *Hyperventilation Syndrome: Research and Clinical Treatment (Johns Hopkins Series in Contemporary Medicine and Public Health)*. 1st ed. (Baltimore, MD: The Johns Hopkins University Press, 1986).

13. Lee et al., "Mouth Breathing, 'Nasal Disuse' and Pediatric Sleep-Disordered Breathing," *Sleep Breath* 4 (2015): 1257-64, doi: 10.1007/ s11325-015-1154-6. Madronio et al., "Older Individuals Have Increased Oro-Nasal Breathing During Sleep," *European Respiratory Journal* 24, no. 1 (2004): 71–77. Gargaglioni et al., "Sex Differences in Breathing," *Comparative Biochemistry and Physiology Part A: Molecular & Integrative Physiology* (2019): 110543.

Chapter 5: Holding Your Breath

1. Michael J. Stephen, M.D., *Breath Taking: The Power, Fragility, and Future of Our Extraordinary Lungs* (New York: Atlantic Monthly Press, 2021).

2. Bohr et al., "Ueber einen in biologischer Beziehung wichtigen Einfluss, den die Kohlensäurespannung des Blutes auf dessen Sauerstoffbindung übt," *Skandinavisches Archiv Für Physiologie* [*Scandinavian Archives of Physiology*] 16.2 (1904): 402-412.

3. *Hatha Yoga Pradipika: The Original Sanskrit by Svatmarama*, 2.2 (trans. Brian Dana Ackers), (Woodstock, NY: YogaVidya.com, 2002).

Chapter 7: Identifying Dysfunctional Breathing

1. Kiesel et al., "Development of a Screening Protocol to Identify Individuals with Dysfunctional Breathing," *International Journal of Sports Physical Therapy* 12, no. 5 (October 2017): 774–786.

2. Patrick McKeown, *The Oxygen Advantage: Simple, Scientifically Proven Breathing Techniques to Help You Become Healthier, Slimmer, Faster, and Fitter* (New York: William Morrow, 2016).

3. Beverly H. Timmons and Ronald Leh, eds., *Behavioral and Psychological Approaches to Breathing Disorders* (New York: Springer, 1994).

4. Bradley and Esformes, "Breathing Pattern Disorders and Functional Movement," *International Journal of Sports Physical Therapy*, 9 no. 1 (February 2014): 28–39.

5. Bordoni et al., "The Anatomical Relationships of the Tongue with the Body System," *Cureus* 10, no. 12 (2018): e3695, https://doi.org/10.7759/cureus.3695.

6. Dr. Steven Lin, *The Dental Diet: The Surprising Link between Your Teeth, Real Food, and Life-Changing Natural Health* (New York: Hay House, 2018). Also, see: Gustafson et al., "Oral and Systemic Effects of Breathing Patterns: Nasal Breathing vs. Mouth Breathing," *Dental Academy of Continuing Education*, https://dentalacademyofce.com/courses/oral-and-systemic-effects-of-breathing-patterns-nasal-breathing-vs-mouth-breathing.

7. Belisa Vranich and Brian Sabin, *Breathing for Warriors: Master Your Breath to Unlock More Strength, Greater Endurance, Sharper Precision, Faster Recovery, and an Unshakable Inner Game* (New York: St. Martin's Essentials, 2020).

8. Mahmood et al., "The Framingham Heart Study and the Epidemiology of Cardiovascular Disease: A Historical Perspective," *Lancet* 383, no. 9921 (March 15, 2014): 999–1008, doi: 10.1016/S0140-6736(13)61752-3.

Chapter 8: Breathing for Daily Life

1. Joseph et al., "Slow Breathing Improves Arterial Baroreflex Sensitivity and Decreases Blood Pressure in Essential Hypertension," *Hypertension* 46, no. 4 (October 2005): 714–8, doi: 10.1161/01.

Chapter 9: Breathing for Sleep

1. Besedovsky, Lange, and Born, "Sleep and Immune Function," *Pflügers Archiv* 463, no. 1 (January 2012): 121–37, doi: 10.1007/s00424-011-1044-0.

2. Matthew Walker, *Why We Sleep: Unlocking the Power of Sleep and Dreams* (New York: Scribner, 2016).

3. Mayo Clinic, "Obstructive Sleep Apnea," Mayo Foundation for Medical Education and Research, accessed September 29, 2023, https://www.mayoclinic.org/diseases-conditions/obstructive-sleep-apnea/symptoms-causes/syc-20352090. National Institute of Health, "What Is Sleep Apnea?" National Heart, Lung, and Blood Institute, accessed September 29, 2023, https://www.nhlbi.nih.gov/health-topics/sleep-apnea.

4. Leah Lagos, *Heart Breath Mind: Conquer Stress, Build Resilience, and Perform at Your Peak* (Boston: Harvest, 2021).

5. Vierra, Boonla, and Prasertsri, "Effects of Sleep Deprivation and 4-7-8 Breathing Control on Heart Rate Variability, Blood Pressure, Blood Glucose, and Endothelial Function in Healthy Young Adults," *Physiological Reports* 10, no. 13 (July 2022): e15389, doi: 10.14814/phy2.15389.

Chapter 10: Breathing for Exercise

1. Svensson, Olin, and Hellgren, "Increased Net Water Loss by Oral Compared to Nasal Expiration in Healthy Subjects," *Rhinology*. 44, no. 1 (March 2006): 74–77.

2. Ortiz Jr. et al., "A Systematic Review on the Effectiveness of Active Recovery Interventions on Athletic Performance of Professional-, Collegiate-, and Competitive-Level Adult Athletes," *Journal of Strength Conditioning Research* 33, no. 8 (August 2019): 2275–2287, doi: 10.1519/JSC.0000000000002589. Dupuy et al., "An Evidence-Based Approach for Choosing Post-exercise Recovery Techniques to Reduce Markers of Muscle Damage, Soreness, Fatigue, and Inflammation: A Systematic Review With Meta-Analysis," *Frontiers in Physiology* 9 (2018 Apr 26): 403, doi: 10.3389/fphys.2018.00403. Dawson et al., "Examining the Effectiveness of Psychological Strategies on Physiologic Markers: Evidence-Based Suggestions for Holistic Care of the Athlete," *Journal of Athletic Training* 49, no. 3 (2014 May-Jun): 331–7, doi: 10.4085/1062-6050-49.1.09. Zope, "Sudarshan Kriya Yoga: Breathing for Health," *International*

Journal of Yoga, 6, no. 1 (January 2013): 4–10, doi: 10.4103/0973-6131.105935. Buchheit, Laursen, and Ahmaidi, "Parasympathetic Reactivation After Repeated Sprint Exercise," *American Journal Physiology Heart Circulatory Physiology* 293, no. 1 (July 2007): H133–41, doi: 10.1152/ajpheart.00062.2007.

3. Elissa Epel, Ph.D., *The Stress Prescription: 7 Days to More Joy and Ease* (New York: Penguin Books, 2022).

4. Martarelli et al., "Diaphragmatic Breathing Reduces Exercise-induced Oxidative Stress," *Evidence-Based Complementary and Alternative Medicine* (2011): 932430, https://doi.org/10.1093/ecam/nep169.

5. Michael J. Stephen, M.D., *Breath Taking: The Power, Fragility, and Future of Our Extraordinary Lungs* (New York: Atlantic Monthly Press, 2021).

6. Bernardi et al., "Acute Fall and Long-Term Rise in Oxygen Saturation in Response to Meditation," *Psychophysiology* 54, no. 12 (December 2017): 1951–1966. doi: 10.1111/psyp.12972. Epub 2017 Aug 25. PMID: 28840941.

Chapter 11: Breathing for Meditation

1. Dr. Andrew Weil, *Breathing: The Master Key to Self-Healing* (Boulder, CO: Sounds True, 2001).

2. Jon Kabat-Zinn, Ph.D., *Full Catastrophe Living: Using the Wisdom of Your Body and Mind to Face Stress, Pain, and Illness* (New York: Bantam, 2013).

3. Zaccaro and Penazzi, "Neurophysiological Model of Altered States of Consciousness Induced by Breathing Techniques," *Cosmos and History* 15 (2019): 200–209. Yadav and Mutha, "Deep Breathing Practice Facilitates Retention of Newly Learned Motor Skills," *Scientific Reports* 6 (November 14, 2016): 37069, doi: 10.1038/srep37069.

4. Melnychuk et al., "Coupling of Respiration and Attention Via the Locus Coeruleus: Effects of Meditation and Pranayama," *Psychophysiology*, 55 (2018): 9.

5. James Mallinson and Mark Singleton, *Roots of Yoga* (New York: Penguin Books, 2017).

6. Ramana Maharshi, *The Collected Works of Ramana Maharshi* (ed. Arthur Osborne) (York Beach, ME: Samuel Weiser, 1997).

Chapter 12: Letting Go with the Breath

1. Frank Ostaseski, *The Five Invitations: Discovering What Death Can Teach Us about Living Fully* (New York: Flatiron Books, 2019).

2. Tsong Khapa, *The Great Treatise on the Stages of the Path to Enlightenment (Volume 1)*, (trans. Lamrim Chenmo Translation Committee) (New York: Snow Lion, 2012).

3. Savanta Group, "Dying Matter Death and Dying Survey," May 15, 2011, carried out by Dying Matters Coalition and poll done by ComRes, accessed September 29, 2023, https://savanta.com/knowledge-centre/poll/dying-matters-death-and-dying-survey-3/.

4. Chagdud Tulku Rinpoche, *Life in Relation to Death* (Junction City, CA: Padma Publishing, 1987).

5. Pew Research Center, "End-of-Life Decisions: How Americans Cope," accessed September 29, 2023, www.pewresearch.org/social-trends/2009/08/20/end-of-life-decisions-how-americans-cope/.

6. Dr. L.S. Dugale, M.D., *The Lost Art of Dying: Reviving Forgotten Wisdom* (New York: HarperOne, July 2021).

7. Rollo May, *Love and Will* (New York: W. W. Norton & Co. Inc., 1969).

Chapter 13: Breathing Your Last Breath

1. Brian Muraresku, *The Immortality Key: The Secret History of the Religion with No Name* (New York: St. Martin's Press, 2020).

2. Lisel Mueller, *Alive Together: New and Selected Poems* (Baton Rouge, LA: LSU Press, 1996). Marcus Aurelius, *Meditations* (trans: Gregory Hays translation) (New York: Random House, 2003).

3. Xu et al. "Surge of Neurophysiological Coupling and Connectivity of Gamma Oscillations in the Dying Human Brain," *Proceedings of the National Academy of Sciences* 120, no. 19 (May 9, 2023): e2216268120, doi: 10.1073/pnas.2216268120.

4. Masel, Schur, and Watzke, "Life Is Uncertain. Death Is Certain. Buddhism and Palliative Care," *Journal of Pain and Symptom Management* 44, no. 2 (August 2012): 307–12. doi: 10.1016/j.jpainsymman.2012.02.018. Delgado-Guay et al., "Spirituality, Religiosity, and Spiritual Pain in Advanced Cancer Patients," *Journal of Pain and Symptom Management* 41, no. 6 (June 2011): 986–94, doi: 10.1016/j.jpainsymman.2010.09.017. Winkelman et al., "The Relationship of Spiritual Concerns to the Quality of Life of Advanced Cancer Patients: Preliminary Findings," *Journal of Palliative Medicine* 14, no. 9 (September 2011): 1022–8, doi: 10.1089/jpm.2010.0536.

5. Frank Ostaseski, *The Five Invitations: Discovering What Death Can Teach Us about Living Fully* (New York: Flatiron Books, 2019).

6. Viktor Frankl, *Yes to Life: In Spite of Everything* (Boston, MA: Beacon Press, 2021).

Chapter 14: Each Breath Is an Opportunity to Begin Again

1. Simone Weil, *First and Last Notebooks* (Oxford: Oxford University Press, 1970).

FURTHER READING

Alua Arthur, *Briefly Perfectly Human: Making an Authentic Life by Getting Real about the End* (Boston: Mariner Books, 2024).

Blandine Calais-Germain, *Anatomy of Breathing* (Seattle: Eastland Press, 2006).

L.S. Dugale, M.D., *The Lost Art of Dying: Reviving Forgotten Wisdom* (New York: HarperOne, 2021).

Elissa Epel, Ph.D., *The Stress Prescription: 7 Days to More Joy and Ease* (New York: Penguin Books, 2022).

Victor Frankl, *Man's Search for Meaning* (Boston: Beacon Press, 2014).

Richard Freeman, *Yoga Breathing: Guided Instructions on the Art of Pranayama* (Boulder, CO: Sounds True, 2014).

David Garrigues, *Vayu Siddhi: A Guide to Pranayama, Ashtanga Yoga's Fourth Limb* (Philadelphia: BookBaby, 2015).

Jon Kabat-Zinn, Ph.D., *Full Catastrophe Living: Using the Wisdom of Your Body and Mind to Face Stress, Pain, and Illness* (New York: Bantam, 2013).

Leah Lagos, *Heart Breath Mind: Conquer Stress, Build Resilience, and Perform at Your Peak* (Boston: Harvest, 2021).

Stephen Levine, *A Year to Live: How to Live This Year As If It Was Your Last* (Washington, DC: Bell Tower, 1998).

Robert Litman, *The Breathable Body: Transforming Your World and Your Life, One Breath at a Time* (Carlsbad, CA: Hay House, 2023).

Gregor Maehle, *Pranayama: The Breath of Yoga* (Adelaide, Australia: Kaivalya Publication, 2012).

James Mallinson and Mark Singleton, *Roots of Yoga* (New York: Penguin Books, 2017).

Patrick McKeown, *Sleep with Buteyko: Stop Snoring, Sleep Apnea and Insomnia, Suitable for Children and Adults* (Moycullen, Ireland: Buteyko Books, 2011).

Patrick McKeown, *The Oxygen Advantage: The Simple, Scientifically Proven Breathing Techniques for a Healthier, Slimmer, Faster and Fitter You* (New York: William Morrow, 2015).

Jill Miller, *Body by Breath: The Science and Practice of Physical and Emotional Resilience* (Las Vegas: Victory Belt Publishing, 2023).

James Nestor, *Breath: The New Science of a Lost Art* (New York: Riverhead Books, 2020).

Frank Ostaseski, *The Five Invitations: Discovering What Death Can Teach Us about Living Fully* (New York: Flatiron Books, 2019).

Matteo Pistono, *Meditation: Coming to Know Your Mind* (Carlsbad, CA: Hay House, 2018).

Stephen Porges, *The Polyvagal Theory: Neurophysiological Foundations of Emotions, Attachment, Communication, and Self-regulation* (New York: W. W. Norton & Company, 2011).

Ramana Maharshi (ed. Arthur Osborne), *The Collected Works of Ramana Maharshi* (York Beach, ME: Samuel Weiser, 1997).

Seneca, *Letters from a Stoic* (trans: Robert Campbell) (New York: Penguin Books, 1969).

Emma Seppälä, *The Happiness Track: How to Apply the Science of Happiness to Accelerate Your Success* (San Francisco: HarperOne, 2017).

Belisa Vranich and Brian Sabin, *Breathing for Warriors: Master Your Breath to Unlock More Strength, Greater Endurance, Sharper Precision, Faster Recovery, and an Unshakable Inner Game* (New York: St. Martin's Essentials, 2020).

Matthew Walker, *Why We Sleep: Unlocking the Power of Sleep and Dreams* (New York: Scribner, 2016).

Dr. Andrew Weil, *Breathing: The Master Key to Self-Healing* (Boulder, CO: Sounds True, 2001).

Florence Williams, *The Nature Fix: Why Nature Makes Us Happier, Healthier, and More Creative* (New York: W. W. Norton & Company, 2017).

INDEX

NOTE: Page references in *italics* refer to figures.
Page references with "n" refer to footnotes.

Index

E

F

G

H

I

Index

Index

Index

IN GRATITUDE

My breath journey began over 30 years ago in the forest surrounding Pashupatinath Temple in Kathmandu, Nepal, where Yogi Bharat introduced me to pranayama and the power of conscious breath holding. That yogic journey continued on both sides of the Himalayas and beyond. Two teachers, Emil Wendel and David Garrigues, profoundly influenced my understanding of the connection between the breath and our vital force, and the profundity of resting in *kevala kumbhaka*. With hands folded, I offer my deep thanks to the three of you, and all yogis who've come before.

Ani Karin at Kopan Monastery in Nepal was my first meditation teacher, and I can't thank her enough for the patience and kindness she offered. Lama Zopa Rinpoche and Khenpo Konchok at Kopan, Geshe Tashi Tsering in London, and Chagdud Rinpoche in the U.S., all urged me in different ways to discover the power of the most subtle breath, and they inspired my inquiry into what happens when our breath ceases. Thank you for your precious teachings on preparing for death.

When I ventured to Tibet, I studied and practiced with a handful of teachers over the course of a decade, for which I'm eternally grateful. Khenpo Jikme Phuntsok and Tashi Gyaltsen Rinpoche initiated and instructed me in the Tibetan Buddhist practice of *tummö*, as well as other esoteric practices. And to the nuns, monks, and pilgrims at mountain hermitages in Nyarong and Derge who offered me a hut and hot meals during my months of retreats—may you find liberation in this lifetime.

Along the sacred Bagmati and Ganges Rivers and in the ashrams in Dharamsala, Goa, and Kerala, I breathed and meditated alongside fellow practitioners who've inspired my journey. This includes meditators at the various Vipassana retreat centers, fellow pujaris in Kathmandu, including Machik Rinpoche and Frances Howland, and the yogis at Satsanga, including Emil, Anouk Aoun, Carroll Dunham, Thomas Kelly, Vidya Roa, and Phil Ernst Lemke. A bow of thanks for the spiritual kinship as we continue our pilgrimage toward the indescribable.

When I returned to the U.S. after many years in Nepal, Tibet, and France, Keith Moore and Casey Craig encouraged me to teach pranayama and meditation; thanks for your support. And to my D.C. yogi meditators, including Kelly Welch, Kate Yonkers, Alice Weil, Marni Kravitz, Jessica Lusty, Joshua Cogan, John and Caroline Osborne, Robb Duncan, Violeta Edelman, and everyone at the Ashtanga Yoga Studio, thanks for your inspiration.

My approach to philosophical inquiry was shaped during my master's degree at the School of Oriental and African Studies (SOAS) at the University of London under Professor Alexander Piatigorsky. He encouraged me to extract a lived experience from the ancient texts and was the first to teach me about *memento mori*, encouraging me to meditate in charnel grounds and cemeteries. Thank you and may your eccentric instructions continue to reverberate.

This book would not have manifested had it not been for the encouragement, insights, and wise counsel from my friends, including Lodi Gyari Rinpoche, Venerable Matthieu Ricard, Sulak Sivaraksa, Roshi Joan Halifax, Sharon Salzberg, Lama Karma Tenzin Choephel, Gary Snyder, Hubert Decleer, Arnie Kotler, Gita Kumar, Eric Weiner, the DeGioia family, Cindy Lee, Natalié Baker, Somboon Chungprampree,

Victoria Sterkin, Mindy Pelz, Ellen Wong, Judd Rogers, Daymond Hoffman, Brot Coburn, Josh Horowitz, Sam Whiting, Michelle Anise, Betty Parsons, and S.K. Pondichery. May everyone find deep spiritual friendship!

And for your healing guidance in Peru's jungle and the crystal caves of Chile, thank you Alberto Villoldo, Marcela Lobos, Spring Washam, Bharath Krishnaswami, Helaine de Grange, and Antonella Velásquez.

Thanks to Oxygen Advantage founder Patrick McKeown, and teachers David Jackson and Anastasis Tzanis for the training to become an Advanced Instructor.

After my wife and I moved to Southern California five years ago, I've been grateful for the support of the team at Patagonia Cardiff, including Troy Yasuda, Dave Hopkins, Natalie Klapp, and Brayden Stephenson, and Ed Lewis at Enjoy the Farm. And I've been inspired by the community of pulmonauts at Our Breath Collective, including Reis Paluso, Luke Wientzen, and Daniella DeVarney.

Deep gratitude to Patty Gift for believing in me, and to Reid Tracy, Margarete Nielsen, and Michelle Pilley for supporting my writing and teaching. Big thanks to my editor, Sally Mason-Swaab, Tricia Breidenthal and Nick Welch of the art team, and all the wonderful folks at Hay House.

As always, my mother, Francey, read every draft along the book's journey, for which I'm grateful. The poet James Hopkins and Lorenzo Lietti offered valuable insights for the book, as did Buteyko teacher and friend, Robert Litman. Thank you.

Thanks to my dad, Chico, and my brother, Mike, for lifting that lodgepole pine tree off my back—otherwise, I would not have written this book.

And finally, most of all, to my most stable support and life partner, Monica. Thank you for your unwavering encouragement and boundless love; they mean the world to me.

ABOUT THE AUTHOR

Matteo Pistono, writer and teacher of meditation and conscious breathing, embarked on his spiritual journey over 30 years ago while living in Nepal and Tibet. Informed by his study of Buddhism, Vedanta, and Hatha Yoga, extensive periods of solitary meditation, and pilgrimages across sacred Himalayan landscapes, Matteo offers an engaged approach to ancient wisdom traditions. His books include *Breathe How You Want to Feel*, *Meditation*, and *In the Shadow of the Buddha*, among others. Matteo earned a Masters in Indian Philosophy from the University of London, and his writings have appeared in *The Washington Post*, BBC, *Buddhadharma*, *Tricycle*, *Men's Journal*, *Kyoto Journal*, and *HIMĀL Southasian*.

Breathe and meditate with Matteo at **matteopistono.com**.

Scan Me

Hay House Titles of Related Interest

YOU CAN HEAL YOUR LIFE, the movie,
starring Louise Hay & Friends
(available as an online streaming video)
www.hayhouse.com/louise-movie

THE SHIFT, the movie,
starring Dr. Wayne W. Dyer
(available as an online streaming video)
www.hayhouse.com/the-shift-movie

***

BOUNDLESS KITCHEN: Biohack Your Body & Boost Your Brain
with Healthy Recipes You Actually Want to Eat, by Ben Greenfield

THE BREATHABLE BODY: Transforming Your World and
Your Life, One Breath at a Time, by Robert Litman

GROW A NEW BODY: How Spirit and Power Plant Nutrients
Can Transform Your Health, by Alberto Villoldo

MEDITATION: Coming to Know Your Mind, by Matteo Pistono

YOU ARE MORE THAN YOU THINK YOU ARE: Practical Enlightenment
for Everyday Life, by Kimberly Snyder

All of the above are available at your local bookstore,
or may be ordered by contacting Hay House (see next page).

We hope you enjoyed this Hay House book. If you'd like to receive our online catalog featuring additional information on Hay House books and products, or if you'd like to find out more about the Hay Foundation, please contact:

Hay House LLC, P.O. Box 5100, Carlsbad, CA 92018-5100
(760) 431-7695 or (800) 654-5126
www.hayhouse.com® • www.hayfoundation.org

———

Published in Australia by:
Hay House Australia Publishing Pty Ltd
18/36 Ralph St., Alexandria NSW 2015
Phone: +61 (02) 9669 4299
www.hayhouse.com.au

Published in the United Kingdom by:
Hay House UK Ltd
The Sixth Floor, Watson House,
54 Baker Street, London W1U 7BU
Phone: +44 (0) 203 927 7290
www.hayhouse.co.uk

Published in India by:
Hay House Publishers (India) Pvt Ltd
Muskaan Complex, Plot No. 3,
B-2, Vasant Kunj, New Delhi 110 070
Phone: +91 11 41761620
www.hayhouse.co.in

———

Access New Knowledge.
Anytime. Anywhere.

Learn and evolve at your own pace
with the world's leading experts.

www.hayhouseU.com